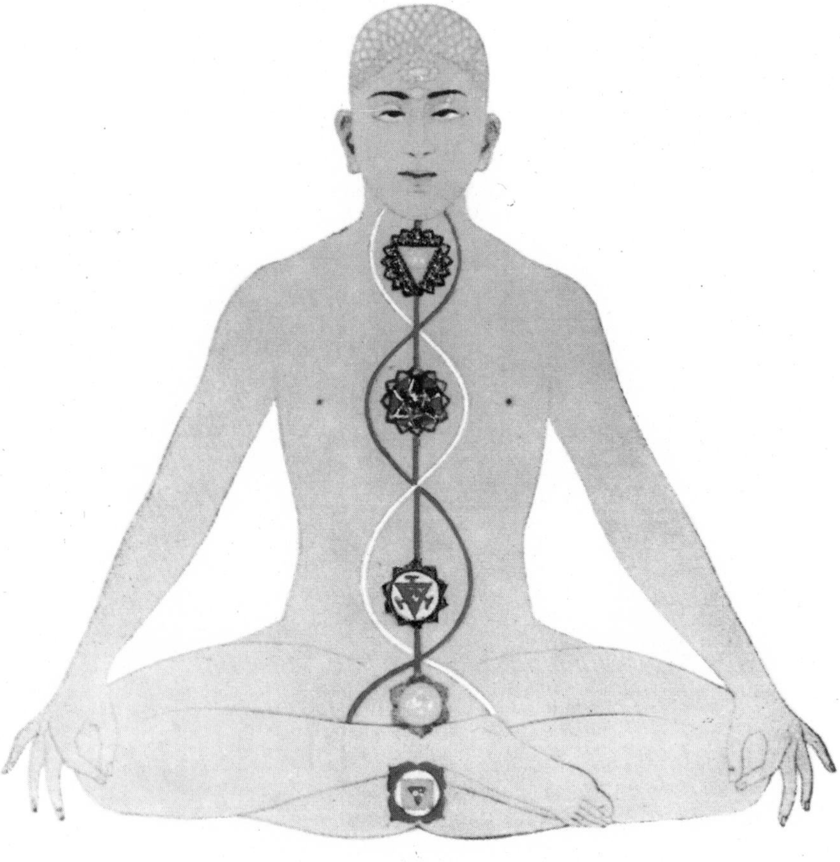

The Centres or Lotuses

Frontispiece

KUNDALINI YOGA

A Brief Study of Sir John Woodroffe's *"The Serpent Power"*

M. P. PANDIT

LOTUS LIGHT PUBLICATIONS
Box 325, Twin Lakes, WI 53181
USA

2nd U.S. edition February 21, 1993

Published by Lotus Light Publications by arrangement
with Sri M.P. Pandit

ISBN 0-941524-50-7
Library of Congress Catalog Card Number 79-88734

Printed in India at All India Press, Pondicherry
for Lotus Light Publications

CONTENTS

PREFATORY

ONE of the most important arrivals in the world of books of late is *The Serpent Power* by Sir John Woodroffe. Now running into its sixth edition, under the sponsorship of the renowned firm *Ganesh & Co.*—a name that has become a byword for the publication of authentic Tantra literature—this remarkable book has been deservedly acclaimed as the most successful work of the author. For, here is found an extraordinarily lucid, elegant and yet exhaustive account of one line of India's spiritual tradition and practice *viz.,* the Sādhana of the Tantras with special reference to the mode of Yoga around which its whole philosophy is centred. The author's presentation of the subject attains a mastery and sublimity unequalled in any of his other works. For Sir John, it will be remembered with gratitude, has been the most redoubtable champion of the much-maligned and thoroughly misunderstood Tantra S'āstra of this ancient land and is responsible for a large number of works seeking to disabuse the rational mind of its unthinking prejudices on the subject and to re-establish the Science in its rightful eminence. It is an old story how this hoary tradition dating from the age of the Veda gradually fell into disuse and misuse with the decline in the general vitality of the Indian civilisation and came to be looked upon with suspicion as little more than black magic and sorcery—if not still worse—and shunned by the 'educated' opinion of modern India. Apart from the cobwebs of ignorance that gathered round the tradition of Tāntric worship and ritual in its waning curve, there was created a good deal of prejudice regarding the Hindu religion by Western writers—with an understandable political motive—in the last century. And it was readily swallowed and mouthed by their zealous Indian following, many of whom, continue even today to repeat and propagate the habitual calumny against what is truly a great Tradition, profound in its conception and spiritual in its aim.

It was given to the solitary figure of Sir John Woodroffe, in the early years of this century, to stand up and vindicate this age-old S'āstra of India against all irrational attacks directed against its prostrate figure not only by alien minds who could not enter into the spirit of its thought, but also by an indifferent progeny blind to their precious heritage. Sir John Woodroffe,[1] a man of deep learning, sharp intellect, catholicity of mind and broadness of understanding had an insatiable interest in oriental subjects and whatever time he could spare from his duties as a member of the Indian Judiciary—a position which he filled with distinction—he devoted to the study of Indian Religion and Philosophy. He insisted on knowing and learning things at first hand[2] and readily accepted the lead of indigenous scholarship[3] in

[1] John George Woodroffe was born on December 15th, 1865. Passing out from Oxford he was called to the Bar by the Inner Temple in 1889 and enrolled the next year as an advocate of the Calcutta High Court. He soon made his mark and was appointed as the Tagore Law Professor. He was raised to the High Court Bench in 1904 and during the next eighteen years of his tenure—during which he once officiated as the Chief Justice—he established a reputation for amazing industry, calm judgment and independence of outlook. After retirement he was the Reader in Indian Law for seven years at the University of Oxford.

Woodroffe was knighted in 1915. He passed away in 1936.

[2] It is said that he even took initiation in the Gāyatrī Mantra from a Guru after undergoing the rituals in the orthodox fashion at Banaras and wore the *yajñopavīta*, the sacred thread. He firmly believed that there was a profound meaning in each aspect of the Hindu Ritual and exerted himself in fathoming it to the core.

[3] His admirable attitude in this matter is best summed up in his own words: "It is necessary to study the Hindu commentators and to seek the oral aid of those who possess the traditional interpretation of the S'āstra. Without this and an understanding of what Hindu worship is and means, absurd mistakes are likely to be made. As regards the Tantra, the great Sādhana S'āstra, nothing which is both of an understanding and accurate character can be achieved without a study of the original texts undertaken with the assistance of the Tāntrik gurus and pundits who are the authorised custodians of its tradition". *(Hymns to the Goddess)*.

matters which were a sealed book to the western mind. He specialised in the study of Tantra S'āstra, particularly the S'ākta System. He was nothing if not thorough: he not only studied, but wherever possible proceeded to convince himself of the practical truth of the Thought. And it was only after he had delved into the arcana of this many-ranged Science and was himself convinced of its genuine worth that he yoked the capacities of his soul and mind in the service of the Tantra. In this task he was ably assisted by his devoted wife, Ellen Woodroffe. He collected valuable manuscripts, edited them, translated them with the help of Indian scholars,[1] prepared introductions and notes, wrote expository treatises and sponsored their publication and circulation with all the authority and prestige that attached to his social and official status.[2] He espoused the cause of Indian culture and spirituality in his lectures and writings and defended it against attacks of the Western critics with rare insight and incisive logic. Doubtless he got unpopular for this with a section of

[1] A fact which he was very scrupulous in acknowledging. In fact he made it a point to use his own name only when the work was entirely his; where he derived active help and collaboration from others he used his nom-de-plume Arthur Avalon. (*Arthur*, it may be mentioned, stands for the perfect knight of traditional British chivalry and *Avalon* is the Valhalla of Celtic heroes).

[2] The more important among these works are:

Introduction to Tantra S'āstra
S'akti and S'ākta
Garland of Letters
The World as Power
Mahāmāya
The Serpent Power
The Great Liberation
Principles of Tantra

For a complete list of these publications the reader may refer to the pages at the end of this book. Many of these works were out of print for a long time. But thanks to the laudable spirit of service and enterprise of the proprietors of *Ganesh and Co.*, we have to-day excellent editions of all of them in a uniform series, with a printing and get-up of the first order. We learn the author had intended to publish works on Hindu Ritual, Sādhana, Philosophy of Yoga, etc. but somehow it was not done.

his own countrymen[1] but he had ultimately the satisfaction of seeing his efforts markedly contributing to the gradual awakening among the educated section of Indians to a proper appreciation of the value of their cultural and spiritual heritage.

He observes somewhere that to understand and expound anything of the profound science of Indian religion and spirituality, one must first place himself in the Hindu skin. We may remark that for Sir John, there was no special need to do so. For the one thing that strikes a close reader of his exposition is that he is truly an Indian soul in a European body. We are not aware if there has been any other non-Indian writer who has succeeded so gloriously in presenting the doctrines and practices of ancient India in terms of modern thought in such a felicitous manner and language as Sir John. The spirit of the original Thought in Sanskrit drips through his transparent writing with a freshness that is invigorating. He lived for three decades in India and developed a deep feeling for the country about which he observes:

"Here man, who has not known himself and his greatness seems nought, and Nature all, a feeling which deepens as night falls on the earth with quick assault, the dark dome

[1] *Vide* some of their press comments:

"It is rather unusual to find among the British members of the Indian Judiciary an apologist for the claims of the Neo-Hindu revivalists and their allies the Extreme Nationalists. It is in this role that we find Sir John Woodroffe figuring as a sort of modern Saul among the prophets". *(Madras Mail)*.

"From keen irritation and annoyance. . . . we passed to a feeling of contempt touched by a sorry sense of amusement. We consider both Mr. Archer and Sir John Woodroffe in this episode a nuisance. . . . There is an absence of clearness even of logic." . . . . (Prof. A Widgery in *The Indian Philosophical Review*).

"Réchauffé of more or less familiar arguments—without the illumination of any new thought—vague, obscure—illogical antithesis and loose and disingenuous assertions –Extravagant abstraction. . . . unable to distinguish form from reality—Vapourising, nebulous . . *(Englishman)*.

of heaven sparkling with the light of countless rising stars, fading again at Dawn as the Visible Devatā, the resplendent joyous Sun, the Eye of Viṣṇu, arises from out the Eastern Mountain. Such a vast scene is but one of many in this, itself vast, secular, and awe-inspiring land. Such a view, we may imagine, was displayed before the eyes of the incoming Āryan peoples. Upon them the influence of the *Soil* fell, filling them with awe. The Spirit, manifesting in this Sacred Earth, at length revealed Itself in their minds. Within them arose the Inner Sun, which is the Light of all, unveiling to the eye of mind truths hidden in its subtle garb of thought. These tenuous veils again fell away, when, by the intuition of the forest-sages, was realised the Spiritual Ether of Consciousness, whose Mother-Power (S′aki) as Will, Thought and Action ever personalises as the life of this magnetic stretch of earth which is India, as the world of which it is an head-ornament, and as (in the words of the Indian Scripture) the countless other universes, which are but the dust of Her Sovereign Feet."[1]

The Serpent Power

This work was first brought out by Sir John Woodroffe in 1918. It is devoted to a detailed exposition of the existence and working of the Six Vital Centres in the human body, the primal Power, Kuṇḍalinī S′akti, lying latent at the base in the system and the process by which it is awakened and speeded upwards piercing through these Centres to reach its destination in the *Sahasrāra* at the crown of the head, achieving thereby the liberation of the individual *jīva* in the infinitude of the Supreme *Siva*. The author has built the work round two original treatises in Sanskrit: (1) *Ṣaṭ Cakra Nirūpaṇa*—description of and investigation into the six bodily

[1] *Sākti and S′ākta* (Preface to the first Edition).

centres. This work in fact forms part, the sixth *Prakāśa*, of a larger work *S'rī Tattva Cintāmaṇi*,[1] by a well-known adept in the Tantras, S'rī Pūrṇānanda Swāmi of Bengal who lived in the middle of the 16th century.

(2) A text called *Pāduka Pañcaka* (Fivefold Footstool of the Guru) celebrating a significant twelve-petalled lotus within the pericarp of the Lotus of thousand petals described in the previous work. It is ascribed to Lord S'iva and so there is no human authorship on record.

Both the works have been here published in Sanskrit with the commentary of Kālīcarana. The original text and the commentary are translated by Sir John Woodroffe who has added notes of his own, drawing points from the commentary of S'aṅkara (not the Ācārya of that name) and

[1] Pūrnānanda who lived now more than four hundred years ago, was a reputed Tāntric sādhaka of high attainments. He was a disciple of Brahmānanda Saraswatī, the commentator of *Advaitasiddhi* and naturally strove to harmonise the teachings of the Vedānta and Tantra in his works. Kālīcarana Siddhānta who came two hundred years later commented upon almost all the works of Pūrnānanda. It is presumed he commented on the whole of *S'rī Tattva Cintāmaṇi*, though only the commentary on the sixth chapter, *S'aṭ Cakra Nirūpaṇa*, has been found and made available.

The *S'ri Tattva Cintāmaṇi*, composed in 1577 A.D., is a voluminous treatise on Tāntric Ritual. Divided into 26 chapters it covers a very wide, almost encyclopaedic range. It may be useful to list here the contents of the work:

1. Note on knowledge and its character. 2. Consecration or Initiation. 3. Places for Initiation, etc. 4. Construction of building (edifice) for the Deity. 5. Subsidiary duties relevant to Initiation. 6. Exposition of the Six Cakras in the body. 7. Characteristics of the Pool (Well) consecrated for the ritual. 8. Offering of oblations to Gods. 9. Varying results of oblations depending upon the things offered. 10. Differences in Mantras. 11. Different S'aktis. 12. Different Mantras. 13. Account of the Soḍaśī Deity. 14 Morning duties. 15. Order of ablutions. 16. Inner sacrifice; Process of creation. 17. S'rī Cakra. 18. Worship of Deity. 19. Hymn to Tripurasundari. 20. Chanting of the Name of Deity to the accompaniment of burnt offerings. 21. Expiatory rites for brahminicide 22. Jñānaduti sacrifice. 23. Revival of the Deity Tripurasundari. 24. Investigation into the reading of Hymns to the Deity. 25. Thousand Names of Tripurasundari. 26. Consecration of Mahāyantra (Mystical Diagram).

This work came to be finally published in full in 1936 under the *Calcutta Sanskrit Series*.

Viśvanātha. As usual, he is at his best in his Notes which always anticipate the difficulties of the modern reader and are to the point. There is, besides, an elaborate Introduction by the learned Editor-Translator running into 350 pages of the most lucid writing explaining the thought-background of the subject-matter of the work, the concepts and the terminology which are peculiar to the Doctrine and Practice that go under the name of Tantra S'āstra.

A number of carefully prepared original coloured plates of the various Cakras, Centres or Lotuses, as described in the text here used, and some half-tone plates showing positions in the Kuṇḍalinī Yoga, included in the volume, go a long way in helping one to assimilate what he reads. The publishers have spared no pains in making the lay-out of the matter as attractive as possible and at the same time ensured its utility to the student by adding indices (both in English and Sanskrit) to half-verses, bibliography and even for words used in the original.

We have had a sense of privilege in handling this magnificent production. The clarity of vision, the mass of knowledge and the rare precision in expression that characterise this noble work have left a deep impression on us. It is to share these gains with like-minded seekers that this brief presentation, in the nature of an introductory hand-book to the larger work, has been undertaken.

S'ri Aurobindo Āśram
Pondicherry
30-3-1959

M. P. PANDIT

INTRODUCTION

In the system of the Tantras there are recognised in the human body certain centres of consciousness, along the spinal column, with their respective spheres of activity. They are six, beginning from the lower end of the spine called the *Mūlādhāra* (foundational support) with an additional seventh at the crown of the head—the *Sahasrāra*. In the lowest bodily centre at the base of the spine, there lies a fundamental Power due to the presence of which the entire organism is enlivened. This Power is described as lying coiled (*kuṇḍalī*) in the Mūlādhāra; it is the *Kuṇḍalī* or *Kuṇḍalinī* S′akti. Coiled in form it is called *Bujangī*, the serpent. This S′akti is a Power of immense potentialities and when activised and set into full and overt operation it can lift man to pinnacles of liberation into Bliss and Knowledge. The Process by which this is brought about by the awakening of the Kuṇḍalinī S′akti is called the Kuṇḍalinī Yoga. It is also called the *Bhūta S′uddhi* as all the elements of the body, the *bhūtas*, are purified as a result of this Yoga.

When roused from its state of rest, the Kuṇḍalī raises its hood as it were and mounts upwards along the spinal column, piercing through all the centres situate in it, 'swallowing' them on its way and reaches its destination at the summit, at the highest centre where awaits her Lord, the S′iva. The effect of this union is an ineffable bliss which pours down into the whole being flooding it with delight.

To be sure, this knowledge of the Cakras or Centres in the body and the latent S′akti does not belong to the Tantras alone.[1] There are references to it in the Yoga

[1] One comes across passages in the Veda touching upon certain yogic phenomena which are described in the Tantras more elaborately, though at times under a dif-

Upaniṣads, in the treatises on Haṭha Yoga. There are even parallels in Sūfi spiritual literature as also in the Māyan (American-Indian) scriptures. Suffice it to say that it figures in one form or another in many of the occult or esoteric systems of ancient communities. This is because it is a fact of organisation in the human body which is come across by every searching enquiry that does not limit itself to the physical appearances. Yet, it is in the Tantras that the Yoga has been worked out so thoroughly; also the stress on acting on the lowest centre to initiate the revolutionary movement is peculiarly Tāntric. So too the location of the chief centres of consciousness along the cerebro-spinal system and in the upper brain. Different systems have placed the chief centres in different parts of the body—some in the breath, some in the blood and some in the heart. In this connection the author cites accounts of the Cakras given by some of the scholars from the West and points out how they err due to a basic failing in their approach: they conceive and describe from a purely materialistic and physiological standpoint whereas the Cakras exist and operate in the subtle body behind the veil of the physical, though the range of their influence and governance extends into the latter. Similarly the author quotes a leading Theosophist, Mr. C. W. Leadbeater, and points out where his reading differs from the Indian systems generally and the Tantra systems in particular, and where lie its weaknesses. Sir John has done well, in this connection, to draw attention to the frequent use of Indian terms by Theosophists but in a sense that is not always the same as given by the Indian and to warn against the inevitable resultant confusion of understanding.

---

ferent nomenclature. S'rī Kapali Sastriar, who combined in himself the best of both the Vedic and the Tāntric disciplines, draws pointed attention to this fact in his writings upon the subject, notably in his commentary on the Ṛg Veda (I Aṣṭaka), the *Siddhāñjana*.

The one chief characteristic that distinguishes the Indian systems, especially the Thought and Practice of the Tantra, is the importance given to *Consciousness*. There are several states of Consciousness and it is the purpose of Yoga to uplift and transform the lower states of Consciousness into the higher.

Put in a nutshell, the central Doctrine that underlies the S′ākta system of the Tantras (on which this work is based) is this. All creation is the manifestation of a Supreme Consciousness. This Consciousness is ineffable and infinite. It spreads itself out in and as Manifestation; yet it is not exhausted by it. The Becoming does not exhaust the Being. It exceeds and stands over it. To put it differently, the Consciousness as Power (that builds the worlds) is supported and based upon Consciousness as Being. The dynamic aspect bases itself on the static. S′akti proceeds from and is sustained by S′iva. This truth of creation holds good everywhere, on the universal scale or on the individual. Man is an expression of this Truth; he holds in himself a central Body-Power which is only partly active in the various modes of the life-energies; there is also in him a fundamental Lord Consciousness which presides over the particular manifestation from its high seat. But the Power is still slumbering with only its superficies in movement. It is lying separated, in effect, from its sustaining base. To emphasise and set into full movement this largely latent Power—the S′akti—and unite it with its Lord is the process of this Yoga which is known by the name of the Primal S′akti, the Kuṇḍalinī. An increasing unfoldment and enlarging expression of the native powers of the manifesting S′akti in the individual frame culminating in a release into the infinitude and the beatitude of its own Highest Status is the goal.

What, then, is this Consciousness that occupies such a central position in this Thought? What is the process of its manifestation?

CHAPTER ONE

CONSCIOUSNESS

THERE is a Supreme Reality which is the ultimate and the irreducible. It is in the nature of a Consciousness, pure and undifferentiated. It is the Cit or *Samvit* which is One everywhere—the Spirit. This Consciousness reveals itself as a S′akti when it manifests as Power. All creation is a product of this Consciousness as Power.

In Theology, the Pure Consciousness is S′iva. His Power is the S′akti—who is one with Him. Both S′iva and S′akti are thus two aspects of the One Reality. It is the same Consciousness that is S′iva-S′akti. S′iva is the static aspect of Consciousness, while S′akti is the active, the kinetic aspect of the same Consciousness. In Vedāntic parlance the same truth is expressed in terms of the Being, *Sat* and the Consciousness, *Cit*, (their common or rather their one nature being Bliss, *Ananda*).

Now, this Consciousness—S′iva-S′akti alone is before all Manifestation. There is first the pure, changeless, static Consciousness, the Para S′iva who in the scheme of the Tattvas or Principles of Creation is termed the *Para Samvit*. Then there is the changing and active aspect of the same which is called the *S′iva-S′akti-Tattva*. Whereas in the *Para Samvit* the state is one of a supreme unitary experience wherein the 'I' and the 'This' are one without distinction, in the *S′iva-S′akti-Tattva* the S′akti "negates Herself as the object of experience leaving the S′iva Consciousness as a mere 'I' not looking towards another." It is the state of subjective illumination (*prakāśa mātra*).

Next the S′akti "presents Herself, but now with the

distinction of 'I' and 'This' as yet held together as part of one self". Here arise the beginnings of Dualism. The Consciousness moves into another station—the *Sadāśiva* or *Sadākhya Tattva* in which the emphasis is laid on the 'This'.

The next state is the *Īśvara-Tattva* where the emphasis is on the 'I' and then follows the third, the *S'uddha-Vidyā-Tattva* where the emphasis is on both, equally. All the while, be it remembered, the whole experience is one; both the aspects or stresses are held in one self. But hereafter, there is a dichotomy. By an operation of the Consciousness which limits itself—called *Māyā*—the united Consciousness is severed: the object 'This' is seen as other than the self 'I' and there follows further separation ensuing in the multiplicity of creation through a graded manifestation of several Tattvas, which are in all computed to be 36 in number.[1]

Viewed from the standpoint of the Mantra S'āstra, this process of Creation, *Sṛṣṭi*, presents itself as follows:

There is the primal *Sakala-S'iva* who is Saccidānanda—corresponding to the S'iva Tattva. From Him proceeds the *S'akti* (S'akti Tattva). From S'akti issues *Nāda* which is the initial movement in the ideating cosmic Consciousness that culminates in the *S'abda-Brahman*—Brahman as Sound. It is the first causal state of what ultimately manifests as

[1] These Tattvas are divided, in the Tantra, into three categories:

(1)	*S'uddha Tattvas* (Pure) :	S'iva Tattva, S'akti Tattva, Sadāśiva Tattva, Īśvara Tattva and S'uddha Vidya Tattva.
(2)	*S'uddha-As'uddha Tattvas* (Pure-Impure) :	Māyā, Five Kañcukas (*Kāla*, *Niyati Rāga*, *Vidyā* and *Kalā*), Puruṣa.
(3)	*As'uddha Tattvas* (Impure) :	Prakṛti, Buddhi or Mahat, Ahaṃkāra, Manas, Five Jñānendriyas, Five Karmendriyas, Five Tanmātras (Sound, Touch, Form, Taste, Odour), Five Elements (Ether, Air, Fire, Water, Earth).

S'abda. (This corresponds to Sadākhya Tattva). From Nāda proceeds the Bindu, rather the *Para Bindu* (Īśvara Tattva). "It denotes that state of active Consciousness or S'akti in which the 'I' or illuminating aspect of Consciousness identifies itself with the total 'This'. It subjectifies the 'This', thereby becoming a point (Bindu) of consciousness with it. When Consciousness apprehends an object as different from Itself, It sees that object as extended in space. But when that object is completely subjectified, it is experienced as an unextended point. This is the universe-experience of the Lord-Experiencer as Bindu."[1]

Both the Nāda and the supreme Bindu are conditions or states of the S'akti in her mood to manifest. The Para Bindu is thus also called the *Ghaṇāvasthā* or the massed state of the S'akti holding in herself all the potentialities of the creation to be. This is the Parama S'iva—The Lord, Īśvara—who holds all the Gods in Himself.

This Para Bindu divides itself into three subsidiary Bindus bringing to the fore its threefold aspect: *Bindu*, *Nāda* and *Bīja*. Of these

(1) *Bindu*, also called the *kārya* (produced) *bindu* to distinguish it from the *Kāraṇa* (causal) *bindu* or Para Bindu, is of the nature of S'iva (*S'ivātmaka*),

(2) *Bīja* of the nature of S'akti,

(3) *Nāda* is S'iva-S'akti—the mutual relation between the S'iva and S'akti.[2]

[1] *The Serpent Power*.

[2] These three Bindus, the Kārya Bindu, the Nāda and the Bīja, are also spoken of as

Para, the transcendent; *Sūkṣma*, the subtle; *Sthūla*, the gross; representing the *Cit*, *Cidacit* and *Acit* aspects of Nature.

They also indicate: (1) the working of the Power of Will, *Icchā*, Knowledge, *Jñāna*, and Action, *Kriyā*.

(2) The Guṇas of *Rajas*, *Sattva* and *Tamas* respectively. They are the manifestations of the Devīs, *Vāmā*, *Jyeṣṭhā* and *Raudrī* and the three Devatas, *Brahmā*, *Viṣṇu* and *Rudra*. The three Bindus are also known as Sun, *Ravi*, Moon, *Candra*,

These three Bindus[1] in their collectivity form the great triangle of *Kāma Kalā*, the Divine Desire for Manifestation. Thus in the language of the Tantras, on the union of S′iva and S′akti (who are truly inseparable), there is a thrill of Nāda; from Nāda is born the Mahā Bindu which again becomes the *Tribindu* (threefold) forming the *Kāmakalā*. Consequent on this threefold bursting of the Supreme Bindu there arise the S′abda Brahman,[2] the Logos, from which issue subsequent formulations of the manifest S′abda and Artha with all their Tattvas and the Lords of Tattvas.

Thus far regarding the creation of the universe which is, as we see, a projection put forth by the S′akti. When the Universe is to be dissolved, it drops back into the S′iva Bindu.[3] The S′akti is conceived as coiling round the S′iva Bindu. This S′akti thus coiled round the S′iva is the *Kuṇḍalinī S′akti.*[4] "She is spoken of as coiled; because She is likened to a serpent (*bhujangī*), which, when resting and sleeping, lies coiled; and because the nature of the power is spiraline, manifesting itself as such in the worlds—the spheroids or 'eggs of Brahma' (*brahmāṇḍa*), and their circular or revolving orbits and in other ways."[5] Now this S′akti coiled round the Supreme S′iva is termed the *Mahā Kuṇḍalī* to distinguish it from the same S′akti in the individual bodies—called the *Kuṇḍalinī*. Just as the Mahā Kuṇḍalī lying around the S′iva (before manifestation) is static potential, similarly the Kuṇḍalinī S′akti in each body is

---

and Fire, *Agni.* It is to be noted that in the first, *i.e.* the Sun, are contained the Fire and Moon and so it is also known as the *Mis′ra-Bindu.*

[1] All the Bindus are indeed the S′akti but each may stress the S′akti or the S′iva aspect it embodies. Thus the white Moon is called the S′iva Bindu and the red Fire is called the S′akti Bindu; the Sun is the mixture of both.

[2] The unmanifested "Sound" which is the source of all manifest S′abda.

[3] Which in its turn is absorbed in the S′iva-S′akti-Tattva anterior to it.

[4] From the word *kuṇḍala*, a coil or a bangle.

[5] *The Serpent Power.*

"the *power at rest* or the *static centre* round which every form of existence as moving power revolves".[1]

Thus, it is the Consciousness which polarises itself into two—the static and the kinetic aspects, the S′iva and the S′akti—that originates and keeps going all Creation. At Dissolution, the Mahā Kuṇḍalī S′akti (which is the Consciousness itself as that S′akti) holds in itself potentially the seed of the next creation, constituted by the collective samskāras or the impressions and tendencies produced by Karma. It is, so to say, the Cosmic Will for manifestation. This seed, when it ripens, awakes the Consciousness into the mood of becoming. "When this seed ripens, S′iva is said to put forth His S′akti. As this S′akti is Himself, it is He in His S′iva S′akti aspect who comes forth (*prasarati*)and endows Himself with all the forms of worldly life. In the pure, perfect, formless Consciousness there springs up the desire to manifest in the world of forms—the desire for enjoyment of and as form. This takes place as a limited stress in the unlimited unmoving surface of pure Consciousness, which is *Niṣkala S′iva*, but without affecting the latter. There is thus change in changelessness and changelessness in change. S′iva in His transcendent aspect does not change but S′iva in His immanent (*sakala*) aspect as S′akti, does. As creative will arises, S′akti thrills as Nāda, and assumes the form of Bindu, which is Īśvara Tattva, whence all the worlds derive. It is for their creation that Kuṇḍalī uncoils. When Karma ripens, the Devī, in the words of the *Nigama*, 'becomes desirous of creation, and covers Herself with Her own Māyā.' Again, 'the Devī, joyful in the mad delight of Her union with the Supreme *Akula*, becomes *Vikāriṇi*'—that is, the *Vikāras* or Tattvas of Mind and Matter, which constitute the universe, appear."[2]

[1] *Ibid.* p. 36.

[2] *The Serpent Power*, pp.38-9.

CHAPTER TWO

CONSCIOUSNESS IN EMBODIMENT

THE same Consciousness which manifests as and in the universe embodies itself also in individual form. The same S'akti is there in man with all its powers; his body is a living storehouse of Power. Yoga aims to raise all the forms of this Power to their highest degree and expression. And the main base, the root of all his powers is the Kuṇḍalinī S'akti.

All form derives from Consciousness as Power. And the Power from which Mind and Matter derive is the Prakṛti-S'akti. The static aspect or the Consciousness in itself as embodied in Mind and Matter is the *Jīvātmā*, the *Puruṣa*.

Prakṛti is the great Matrix of all things born.[1] And Prakṛti is the great Consciousness itself as creative Power. Prakṛti "finitises and makes form in the infinite formless Consciousness." There are three modes, or Guṇas as they are called, in which it functions: first, the mode of revealing the consciousness (*sattva*), second, the mode of activising it (*rajas*) and the third, of veiling it (*tamas*). All the three Guṇas coexist, only with varying stresses. The Guṇa which conceals the Pure Consciousness predominates in the lower scales of Nature whereas the Guṇa which reveals it predominates in the higher scales. The object of Yoga is to develop and intensify the Sattva Guṇa and gain passage to the Pure Consciousness, Cit.

When the Prakṛti is quiescent, that is unmanifest, all the three Guṇas are in an equilibrium. At the moment of creation, there is (owing to the impulsion of the *kārmic*

[1] *Kṛteh prārambho yasyāh* whose is the beginning of creation, *prakṛyate kāryādikam anayā*, by whom is done creation, maintenance and dissolution.

Forces) a stir of the Guṇas, *guṇakṣobha*, and a vibration, *spandana*, issues forth as the original *S'abda Brahman*, Cosmic Sound. The Guṇas move into action, affect each other, and the creation is begun. There appears Form out of the Formless. *Prakṛti* moves into *Vikṛti*, change. These *vikṛtis*, or self-modifications of the Prakṛti are the original *tattvas*, the categories of Mind, Senses and Matter.

The Jīva which is in fact the Consciousness particularised in an individual form, lodges itself in a triple body or in three bodies so to say, all of which are successively evolved from the Prakṛti-S'akti. They are:

(1) The Causal body, *kāraṇa śarīra*, in which the Jivātma lives until it is united with the Paramātma, the Supreme bodiless Spirit. It is in this body that the Jīva poises itself in dreamless sleep.

(2) The subtle body, projected and supported by the causal—is the *sūkṣma* or *linga śarīra* in which the Jīva exists during dreams. The subtle body consists of the first evolutes of the causal *viz.*, the Mind and the Senses and their supersensible objects.[1]

(3) Deriving from the subtle is the gross body, the body of matter, *bhūta*, which is the object of senses derived from the supersensibles. The Jīva lives in this form in the *jāgrat*, the waking state.

It is to be noted that Mind in this system is a broad term embracing in its connotation many forms and modifications of the Prakṛti. Thus it comprises:

Buddhi or *Mahat Tattva* which is simply a consciousness of Being;

Ahaṃkāra, the consciousness realising itself as the particular experiencer, the 'I';

[1] *Antaḥkaraṇa*, internal instrument, *bāhya karaṇa*, external instruments (*Indriyas*), and the *Tanmātras*.

Manas, the desire which arises on the basis of this personalised consciousness;

Indriyas (senses) which are differentiated faculties of the Consciousness for the enjoyment of the experience. They are of two kinds: those of perception (*jnānendriya*) and those of action (*karmendriya*). They are to be distinguished from the sense organs like the ear, eye, tongue etc. which are only the instruments through which the faculties operate.[1]

The senses (Indriyas) require objects for their perceptions, the sensations. And these sense-objects presuppose certain general elements, their parent universals. They are termed *Tanmātras*, the subtle and general elements of sense perceptions which render possible the subsequent sensations of hearing, touch, sight, taste and smell. They are the abstract qualities or universals of Sound (*śabda tanmātra*), Touch (*sparśa tanmātra*), Sight *i.e.,* form (*rūpa tanmātra*), Taste (*rasa tanmātra*) and Odour (*gandha tanmātra*). They are the *sūkṣma bhūtas* from which derive the ordinary or gross *bhūtas* or objects of senses.

The sense objects derived from the Tanmātras strike the Indriyas, the senses, whereupon attention is drawn to them. But there may be a number of sensations at the same time. A particular sensation is selected and gathered by the Manas which in turn refers to the Ahaṃkāra, the I-maker, after which the Buddhi determines, and forms concepts, 'It is so', or resolves 'It must be done'. This Buddhi illumined as it is by the light of Cit (Consciousness) that is the Puruṣa is indeed the principal Tattva which is "the thinking principle

[1] These organs, the author points out, are not always necessary for the faculties to act. Under certain conditions it is possible to dispense with them. So also the faculties could function through organs not specifically made for that purpose. Sir John quotes the case recorded by Prof. Lombroso "of a woman who, being blind, read with the tip of her ear, tasted with her knees and smelt with her toes." (*The Serpent Power*, p. 60).

which forms concepts or general ideas acting through the instrumentality of Ahaṃkāra, Manas and the Indriyas. In the operations of the senses Manas is the principal; in the operation of Manas, Ahaṃkāra is the principal; and in the operation of the Ahaṃkāra, Buddhi is the principal. With the instrumentality of all of these Buddhi acts, modifications taking place in Buddhi through the instrumentality of the sense functions. It is Buddhi which is the basis of all cognition, sensation, and resolves, and makes over objects to Puruṣa, that is, Consciousness. And so it is said that Buddhi, whose characteristic is determination, is the charioteer; Manas, whose characteristic is *saṃkalpavikalpa*, is the reins; and the Senses are the horses. Jīva is the Enjoyer (*Bhoktā*)."[1]

A word may be added about the real nature of *Matter* of which the gross body is formed. The body is composed of a number of compounds which again are formed by a number of elements; further analysis through the molecule and the atom reveals a Primordial Substance of which all else is a modification. This Substance, says modern Science, is the Ether, *ākāśa*. In the Indian theory, however, Ākāśa itself is one of the differentiations of the Primordial Power, the Prakṛti-S'akti—a formulation of the Supreme Consciousness. Matter is thus truly a form of Consciousness.

What is called sensible Matter in the West corresponds to the *Mahābhūtas* produced from the Tanmātras. They are *Ākāśa* (Ether), *Vāyu* (Air), *Tejas* (Fire), *Āpas* (Water) and *Pṛthivī* (Earth). They are described as "five forms of motion into which the Prakṛti differentiates itself".

Each form in this material universe is a product—a compound—of all the Bhūtas. Hence each thing contains the characteristics of all the Bhūtas. That is why the Tantra emphasises that each has its own form, colour, sound—all

[1] *The Serpent Power*, p. 63.

interrelated. Sir John points out that sounds of speech and music have their own forms which are now verifiable by the Phonoscope. "When words are spoken or sung into a small trumpet attached to the instrument, a revolving disk appears to break up into a number of patterns, which vary with the variations in sound."[1] Each Tattva has its own form (*Maṇḍala*) and colour.[2]

Vitalising and sustaining the body is the Life-Force, the *Vāyu*, which is a special expression of the Energy aspect of the Consciousness. As vital *Vāyu*, it courses as the currents of nerve-force. As related to the body, it is called *prāṇa* and works in a fivefold manner in the body—as five *prāṇas* with different locations and functions. Of them the first called *Prāṇa*, (bearing the same name as the Force in its totality) is the breath of life moving in the upper part. It is the function concerned with the intake of the universal Life-Force for distribution inside the organism and its expiration. Prāṇa is located in the heart region. The second is the *Apāna*, the downward breath, situate in the lower trunk, pulling against the Prāṇa. It is in the anus and governs excretory functions. The third is the *Samāna*, governing the interaction and balancing of the above two forces. Located in the navel region it maintains the equilibrium of the vital forces and controls the process of digestion and assimilation. The fourth is the *Vyāna*, which pervades the whole body and distributes the energies and generally holds together the body in all its parts. The fifth and last is the *Udāna*

[1] *The Serpent Power*, p. 71.

[2] Thus *Ākās'a* is denoted by a transparent white circle (with dots),
Vāyu by a smoky grey six-cornered diagram,=
Tejas by a red triangle,
Āpas by a white crescent-shaped diagram,
Pṛthivī by a yellow quadrangular figure.

"Similarly, to each Devata also there is assigned a yantra or diagram which is a suggestion of the form assumed by the evolving Prakṛti or body of that particular Consciousness". *Ibid*, p. 72.

(in the throat), the ascending Vāyu which moves upward from the body to the head and is the channel for reaching the supra-physical planes.[1]

Subsidiary to these five main divisions, there are five minor *Vāyus*. They are *Nāga* (manifest in the hiccup), *Kūrma* (in the opening and closing of the eyes), *Kṛkara* (indigestion), *Devadatta* (in yawning) and *Dhanañjaya* (which is the vāyu active even in the dead body).

We have spoken of the kinds of bodies, the several constituents of the Mind, the functional forms of the Life-Force. It now remains to take into account the states of consciousness as embodied in the Jīva. In itself Consciousness has no states, but when it expresses itself as the being or Jīva, in manifestation, it has three tiers of conditions of existence:

(1) The waking state, *jāgrat*, in which the Jīva is aware of external objects (*bahiprajňa*) and enjoys them through the senses, *sthūla-bhuk*. In this state the Jīva is called the *Jāgari* and the gross body housing this consciousness the *Viśva*. The corresponding state of the Cosmic Jīva (the universal Being) is known as the *Vaiśvānara*.

(2) The dream state, *svapna*, in which the Jīva is aware of internal objects (*antaḥprajña*) and enjoys what is subtle, *pravivikta-bhuk*—the impressions left by the objects experienced in the waking consciousness. Here the Jīva consciousness is in the subtle body and is known as the *Taijasa*. The corresponding state of the collective Being is the *Hiraṇyagarbha*. Sir John Woodroffe adds also the *Sūtrātma* and mentions the distinction between the two *e.g.*, Paramātman manifest as collective *Antaḥkaraṇa* is the Hiraṇyagarbha and as collective *Praṇa* is the Sūtrātma.

[1] "The functions of Prāna may be scientifically defined as follows: Appropriation (Prāna), Rejection (Apāna), Assimilation (Samāna); Distribution (Vyāna) and Utterance (Udāna)." *The Serpent Power*, p. 78.

(3) The state of dreamless sleep, *suṣupti*, in which the Jīva is neither objective, *bahiprajña* nor subjective, *antaḥ-prajña*, but simply gathered in himself—without any object other than himself—*prajñāna ghaṇa.* The Jīva here is called the *Prājña* and lives in the causal, *kāraṇa*, body, which is Prakṛti allied to Consciousness. The corresponding cosmic state is the *Īśvara.* This is the state of Bliss, Ananda; the Jīva here enjoys the Bliss, he is *ānandabhuk.* In the first state the Jīva enjoys the gross objects in the second, the subtle objects; in this the third, he does not enjoy through any kind of objects but seizes Bliss directly without any subject or object. But this *suṣupti* state is not yet Brahman Consciousness, for there is here still the identification with Prakṛti. It is only in the

(4) Fourth state, the *Turīya*, that the Jīva has pure experience called *S'uddha-vidyā.* The Jīva here lives in the great Causal (*Mahā kāraṇa*) body.

Beyond even the fourth, it is said there is a still higher, the transcendent state—the *Turīyātita.* Here are the *Unmeṣa* and *Nimeṣa* states of Consciousness (opening and closing of the Eye of Consciousness) with the *Īśvara Tattva* and the *Sadākhya Tattva* respectively, leading to the final and perfect Śiva Consciousness.

CHAPTER THREE

MANTRA

THE subject of Mantra occupies a key position in this system. In fact Mantra S'āstra is another name for Tantra S'āstra. The Mantra is a syllable or syllables with power. And like all power it can be used for any purpose, good or otherwise. The author cites in illustration a number of different applications *viz.* the communication of spiritual power to the disciple from the Guru by means of Mantra, the lighting up of a Homa Fire by Mantra, elimination of harmful agencies, etc. We might also cite the recorded incident of a well-known yogin in South India who once came across a festive party in the course of his itinerary and joined the celebrations for the nonce. The host, who was not aware of his identity, asked him to grind paste from sandalwood for after-dinner colling use by the guests. He of course obliged and prepared the paste, all the while humming to himself an *agni mantra.* Imagine the consternation of the guest, when later they used the paste only to feel terrific heat on its contact! Obviously the mantra, when chanted by the yogin, had invoked Agni and the paste was pervaded by its physical nature—the fire element.

What is a Mantra? Mantra is a power, it is S'akti in the form of Sound. Sound, *śabda*, is of two kinds: lettered sound, *varṇatmaka*, and unlettered sound, *dhvanyātmaka.* The *dhvani* is caused by the striking of two things together whereas the former is not caused by any striking; it is *anāhata*, not struck. It is independent of this movement and is eternal. The Dhvani manifests it; it is the S'abda that manifests thus that is eternal. The sound, *dhvani*, is produced by the contact of the vocal organ with air as a result of a movement or thought in the mind seeking expression in sound. It is to be noted that sound, *dhvani*, is not the only form in which S'abda finds expression. Besides the auditory, there can be the visual expression as also the tactual expression (*e.g.* perforated dots to the blind).

According to the Indian psychology, when an object, *artha*, comes before the mind for perception, the mind modifies itself (*vṛtti*) into the form of that object. This self-modification of the mind into the shape of the object of perception is the subtle object, *sūkṣma artha*, corresponding to the gross object, *sthūla artha.* Besides the aspect of mind as the perceived (in the self-modified form of the object), there is another and more fundamental, mind as the perceiver; thus mind is at once the cogniser and the cognised, the *grāhaka* and the *grāhya*, the revealer and the revealed, *prakāśaka* and *prakāśya*, the denoter and the denoted, *vācaka* and *vacya.* Now that aspect which cognises is called the *S'abda* or *Nāma* and the aspect in which it becomes the cognised is the *Artha* or *Rūpa.* The outer physical object (of which the mental is an impression) is also the *Rūpa* and the spoken word relevant to it is the (outer) *S'abda.* The entire creation is thus *Nāma* and *Rūpa.*

There are gradations in which the Original Śabda, the Brahman Sound, manifests itself. The first is the state of *Parā*: sound is yet motionless and comes into being on the differentiation of the Mahābindu. In the human body it exists in the Mūlādhāra Centre as motionless causal *S'abda.* This unmanifest *Para S'abda* is the Kuṇḍalī Sakti.

The second state—*Paśyanti*— is one in which the S'abda begins to move, but yet with an undifferentiated and general motion. In the body its place is from Mūlādhāra to the Maṇipūra.

Next is the *Madhyamā* sound, the state in which appear

the subtle Nāma and Rūpa, the activity of the Mind as the cogniser and the cognised takes place. The operation is in the subtle field and the sound is called the *Hiraṇyagarbha S'abda*. In the body it extends from Paśyantī to the heart.

The fourth state is the *Vaikharī* in which the *Madhyamā Śabda* is projected into the gross outer as the *Virāṭ Sabda*. In the body it is the uttered Speech which issues from the throat.

In the words óf the author: "In creation *Madhyamā S'abda* first appeared. At the moment there was no outer *Artha*. Then the cosmic mind projected this inner *Madhyamā Artha* into the world of sensual experience, and named it in spoken speech (*Vaikharī S'abda*). The last or *Vaikharī S'abda* is uttered speech developed in the throat issuing from the mouth. This is *Virāṭ S'abda*. *Vaikharī S'abda* is therefore language or gross lettered sound. Its corresponding *Artha* is the physical or gross object which language denotes. This belongs to the gross body (*Sthūla Śarīra*). *Madhyamā-Śabda* is mental movement or ideation in its cognitive aspect, and *Madhyamā Artha* is the mental impression of the gross object. The inner thought-movement in its aspect as *S'abdārtha*, and considered both in its knowing aspect (*S'abda*) and as the subtle known object (*Artha*), belongs to the subtle body (*Sūkṣma-S'arīra*). The cause of these two is the first general movement towards particular ideation (*Paśyanti*) from the motionless cause, *Para-S'abda*, or Supreme Speech. Two forms of inner or hidden speech, causal and subtle, accompanying mind movement, thus precede and lead up to spoken language. The inner forms of ideating movement constitute the subtle, and the uttered sound the gross, aspect of Mantra, which is the manifested S'abda-Brahman."[1]

[1] *The Serpent Power.*

To put it in brief: when the S'akti moves into Ideation, which is precedent to Creation, She is the *Para-Vāk*. The next state is the *Paśyantī Vāk* in which the *Ichhā S'akti* is about to manifest the world. The third, *Madhyamā-Vāk* is the play of *Jñāna S'akti* when the first form—*Mātṛkā*—is assumed and the first particularised movement takes place. The last—*Vaikhari-Vāk*—state is when the *Kriyā S'akti* projects the gross letters and the gross objects.

Thus uttered speech manifests the inner speech which is idea or thought. It is this inner thought-movement which is an operation of consciousness that is expressed by the outer speech; the uttered word carries behind itself the idea-power of which it is a projection into gross expression. Under proper conditions to utter the word is to evoke this power of consciousness into activity. This in sum is the principle of Mantra.

One point to be noted before we pass further. We spoke of lettered sound—*varṇātmaka śabda*. These letters in which the subtle sound forms itself are not the gross letters of the alphabet we are familiar with. They are subtle and causal forms called *Mātṛkā*. The letters issuing from the throat are gross correspondences of those *Mātṛkās*, just as the spoken *śabda* and the physical object, *artha*, are correspondences of the subtle *śabda* and *artha*.

The Tantra S'āstra allocates particular letters (subtle ones) to particular centres or Cakras in the body. Also in each Cakra there is the seed, *bīja*, mantra of a Tattva. The Tattva evolves from that seed-letter or letters. Thus the Bīja Mantra of a thing is its natural Name. "The natural Name of anything is the sound which is produced by the action of the moving forces which constitute it. He therefore, it is said, who mentally and vocally utters with creative force the natural name of anything, brings into being the thing which bears that name. Thus *'Raṃ' is the Bīja* of fire in the Maṇipūra

Cakra. This Mantra *'Raṃ'* is said to be the expression in gross sound (*Vaikharī S'abda*) of the subtle sound produced by the forces constituting fire. The same explanation is given as regards *'Laṃ'* in the Mūlādhāra, and the other Bījas in the other Cakras."[1]

It is to be noted, however, that mere chanting or repetition of the Mantra cannot be effective. The consciousness in the Mantra, its real power must be awakened, before it can act. Thus to invoke a Devatā which is the object, *artha*, its Name, the *mantra* must be awakened, *prabuddha*; its consciousness, *caitanya*, rendered alive. The author's remarks in this connection are worth quoting:

"The mere utterance, however, of *'Raṃ'* or any other Mantra is nothing but a movement of lips. When, however, the Mantra is 'awakened' (*prabuddha*)—that is, when there is *Mantra-Caitanya* (Mantra-Consciousness)—then the Sādhaka can make the Mantra work. Thus in the case cited the *Vaikhari S'abda*, through its vehicle *Dhvani*, is the body of a power of Consciousness which enables the Mantrin to become the Lord of Fire. However this may be, in all cases it is the creative thought which ensouls the uttered sound which works now in man's small 'magic', just as it first worked in the 'grand magical display' of the World Creator. His thought was the aggregate, with creative power, of all thought. Each man is S'iva, and can attain His power to the degree of his ability to consciously realise himself as such. For various purposes the Devatās are invoked. *Mantra* and *Devatā* are one and the same. A *Mantra-Devatā* is *S'abda* and *Artha*, the former being the name, and the latter the Devatā whose name it is. By practice (Japa) with the Mantra the presence of the Devatā is invoked. Japa or repetition of Mantra is compared to the action of a

[1] *The Serpent Power.*

3

man shaking a sleeper to wake him up. The two lips are are S'iva and S'akti. Their movement is the coition (*maithuna*) of the two. S'abda which issues therefrom is in the nature of Seed or Bindu. The Devatā thus produced is, as it were, the 'son' of the Sādhaka. It is not the Supreme Devatā (for it is actionless) who appears, but in all cases an emanation produced by the Sādhaka for his benefit only."[1]

How to realise the creative power of a Mantra? What is the process to awaken it and the way to use it for the achievement of one's purpose? This knowledge is embodied in the Mantra Vidya.

Again, letters by themselves have no power to reveal any *artha*. There is, prior to all manifest *artha* and *śabda*, a causal undivided state of Brahman consciousness formulated as an undifferentiated, pervasive *S'abda*, the *S'abda-Brahman*. This unmanifest *S'abda*, Sound, is the cause of all *S'abda* and *Artha*. It is the celebrated *S'phoṭa* which discloses the meaning of every word; it awakens the cognition of a thing the moment the word denoting it is uttered. In the human body the *S'abda-Brahman* takes the form of Kuṇḍalinī S'akti and manifests itself in the *letters*[2] at the various centres.

[1] *The Serpent Power.*

[2] There are in all 51 of them; in the language of the S'ākta Tantra the Kuṇḍalinī has 51 coils.

CHAPTER FOUR

CAKRAS

ALL the Tattvas, Cosmic Principles, in Creation are there embedded in the body. Each Tattva, however, has its own centre of activity, the place where it is most preponderant and from where radiate its energisings into the system. These are the locii called, in the Tantras, the Centres or Cakras (Circles). They are not, of course, anatomical locations seizable by the gross eye. They are subtle centres—seats—of consciousness, S'akti, active in the body and are situate within the spinal system beginning from the lower end of the spinal column up to the top of the brain. The range of the activity and influence of each Centre extends to its corresponding region in the gross physical body—the various plexuses and cerebral centres. From each of them radiate thousands of *Nāḍis*, conduits of *prāṇic* force in different directions. These Nāḍis too are not to be confused with the nerves and arteries with which medical science is familiar. They are subtle channels of the vital energies and are visible to the yogic *dṛṣṭi* alone. They are therefore called the *yoga-nāḍis*. It is the configuration of these Nāḍis that gives rise to the appearance of petals of lotuses to each of the Centres which look like so many lotuses, each with a different number of petals.

The principal Nāḍis are said to be fourteen in number.[1] Chief among them, however, are three, *Iḍā*, *Suṣumnā* and the *Pingalā*. Of these three again the Suṣumnā is the most important.

[1] In fact there are computed to be thousands of Nāḍis in the body; but of them only a few, fourteen of them, are important. They are: "1. Suṣumnā, in the central

The Suṣumnā is situated within the spinal column, the *Merudaṇḍa*, in the interior canal; it extends from the Mūlādhāra, the basic plexus, to the twelve-petalled lotus in the pericarp of the thousand-petalled lotus above. Within this Suṣumnā is a subtle Nāḍi, the *Vajriṇī*, and within it a still subtler one, the *Citṛiṇī*. The interior of the Citṛiṇī is called the *Brahma Nāḍi.* It is the channel for the movement of Kuṇḍalinī. It is not a separate Nāḍi in the usual sense, but only a *vivara*, a hollow passage. The opening of this Citriṇī Nāḍi is the door through which the Kuṇḍalinī enters the Royal Road, *Kula Mārga*, on its way to the Lord and it is known as *Brahma-Dvāra.*

To the left of this Nāḍi, on the outside of the Meru, is the Iḍā and to the right is the Piṅgalā. Both of them entwine the Suṣumnā from left to right and right to left in the movement upward going round the Lotuses. These are also known as Ganga (Iḍā), Yamuna (Piṅgalā) and Sarasvati (Suṣumnā). They all meet at the Mūlādhāra and again at

---

channel of the spinal cord. 2. Iḍā, the left sympathetic chain, stretching from under the left nostril to below the left kidney in the form of a bent bow. 3. Pingalā, the corresponding chain on the right. 4. Kuhū, the pudic nerve of the sacral plexus, to the left of the spinal cord. 5. Gāndhāri, to the back of the left sympathetic chain, supposed to stretch from below the corner of the left eye to the left leg. . . . 6. Hastijihva to the front of the left sympathetic chain, stretching from below the corner of the left eye to the great toe of the left foot. . . . 7. Sarasvati, to the right of Suṣumnā, stretching up to the tongue (the hypoglossal nerves of the cervical plexus). 8. Pūśā, to the back of the sympathetic chain, stretching from below the corner of the right eye to the abdomen (a connected chain of cervical and lumbar nerves). 9. Payasvini, between Pūśā and Sarasvati, auricular branch of the cervical plexus on the left. 10. Sankhini between Gāndhāri and Sarasvati, auricular branch of the cervical plexus on the left. 11. Yaśasvini, to the front of the right sympathetic chain, stretching from the right thumb to the left leg (the radial nerve of the brachial plexus continued on to certain branches of the great sciatic). 12. Vārunā, the nerves of the sacral plexus, between Kuhū and Yaśasvinī, ramifying over the lower trunk and limbs. 13. Viśvodarā, the nerves of the lumbar plexus, between Kuhū and Hastijihvā ramifying over the lower trunk and limbs. 14. Alambuṣā, the coccygeal nerves, proceeding from the sacral vertebrae to the urino-genitary organs." (Dr. Brojendranath Seal's account cited by Sir John Woodroffe, *The Serpent Power.*)

the Ājñā Cakra. The meeting place at the Mūlādhāra is the *Yukta Triveṇi*. The Ājñā Cakra where they meet again and form a plaited knot—and enter the Suṣumnā,—is the *Mukta Triveṇi*. Thereafter they separate and flow separately (hence *Mukta Triveṇi*) and proceed in the different nostrils. It may be mentioned that Iḍā is also described as the Moon and Piṅgalā, as the Sun, representing the negative and positive phases of the current activity.

MŪLĀDHĀRA

Midway between the genitals above and the anus below, at the place where the Suṣumnā Nāḍi and the root of all Nāḍis (*Kaṇḍa*) meet, is the first centre, the *Mūlādhāra*[1] *Cakra*. The Mūlādhāra Lotus is the *subtle centre* of this region, within the spinal column, with its head hanging downwards.[2] The colour of this lotus is crimson ; the number of petals is four with the letters *vaṁ*, *śaṁa*, *ṣaṁ* and *saṁ* upon them in gold. Each of these letters is a Mantra, a S'akti and as such a *devatā* attending (*āvaraṇa*) upon the Principal Devatā of the Cakra. All the letters of the Lotuses constitute together the Mantra body of the Kuṇḍalinī S'akti. The Tattva of which this lotus is the centre is the *Pṛthivī*, Earth, whose form is a square and colour yellow and its Bīja (seed) Mantra is *laṁ*. That is to say, *laṁ* is the *vaikharī* sound expressive of the subtle sound produced by the vibration of the particular forces active in this Centre. This Bīja is further described as being seated on Elephant *Airāvata* (the Elephant denoting qualities of the reigning Tattva,

[1] *Mūla* (root), *ādhāra* (support)—is the root of the Suṣumnā which is also the resting place of the Kuṇḍalinī. It is also so called as it is at the root of all the six Cakras.

[2] All the lotuses have their faces turned downwards; they turn upwards only when the Kuṇḍalinī S'akti, moving up, strikes them.

strength, firmness and solidity). The Elephant is also the *vāhana* (vehicle) of Indra whose Seed-Mantra is here.

The Devata of the Centre is the creative Brahmā and his S'akti is Savitrī. There is also here S'akti Dākinī who is the S'akti of the *Dhātu*, bodily substance, of this Centre. She is the revealer of the *Tattva-Jñāna*, knowledge of Tattva.

Further, here is the Yoni, the Triangle—*S'akti Pīṭha*—in which is the S'ivalinga called *Svayambhū* with the shape of a tender leaf. It represents the aspect of Brahman manifested in this Centre; its colour is yellow. "The Devi Kuṇḍalinī, luminous as lightning, shining, in the hollow of this lotus like a chain of brilliant lights, the World-bewilderer who maintains all breathing creatures, lies asleep coiled three and a half times round the Linga, covering with Her head the Brahmadvāra."[1]

SVĀDHIṢTHĀNA

Next above, at the root of the genitals is the *svādhiṣṭhāna Padma*. Unlike the Mūlādhāra which is at the root of the Suṣumnā, this Cakra is placed within the Suṣumnā Nāḍi. This lotus of vermilion colour has six petals, with the letters, *baṁ*, *bhaṁ*, *maṁ*, *yaṁ*, *raṁ* and *laṁ*, shining like lightning. The regnant Tattva of this centre is *Ap*, Water, and hence the Cakra is also known as the white region of Varuṇa (the Deity of the Ocean). The characteristic form or Maṇḍala of this Tattva is the Crescent Moon and the colour white. The Bīja is *vaṁ* and this varuṇa Bīja is seated on a white *Makara* (animal like an alligator) which is the *vāhana* of Varuṇa. The Devatās that preside here are Hari (Viṣṇu) and Rākinī.

[1] *The Serpent Power.*

MAṆIPŪRA

Above this, at the centre of the navel region, is the *Maṇipūra* or the *Nābhi Padma* of dark hue (like the heavy-laden rain clouds), of ten petals with the letters *ḍaṁ*, *ḍhaṁ*, *ṇaṁ*, *taṁ*, *thaṁ*, *daṁ*, *dhaṁ*, *naṁ*, *paṁ*, *phaṁ*, in the colour of blue lotus. The Tattva is Tejas, in fact the *padma* is called Maṇipūra because it is *lustrous* as a gem, *maṇi*, owing to the presence of the Tejas; its form is the triangle and colour red. The red Bīja of Fire *Raṁ* is seated on a ram, the *vāhana* of Agni. Here are God Rudra and S′akti Lākinī.

These are the three Centres from which the *Virāṭ*, the gross body, is formed.

ANĀHATA

Further up, in the heart-region is the Lotus called *anāhata padma*. It is so called because here it is that the yogin first hears the *śabda brahman*, the sound that is produced without the striking of two things together, *anāhata*, which is the usual occasion for any sound. This lotus of the colour of *Bandhūka* flower has ten petals with letters in vermilion, *kaṁ*, *khaṁ*, *gaṁ*, *ghaṁ*, *ngaṁ*, *caṁ*, *chaṁ*, *jaṁ*, *jhaṁ*, *jñaṁ*, *ṭaṁ*, *ṭhaṁ*. This is the abode of the Jīvātman called the *Hamsa*. The Tattva is Vāyu; its region is six-cornered, hexagonal—two triangles with one of them inverted and its colour smoky-grey. The Vāyu Bīja *yaṁ* is seated on a black antelope (whose chief quality is speed), the *vāhana* of Vāyu. Īśa the Overlord of the first three Cakras and S′akti Kākinī are here.

In the downward pointing triangle (which is a form of S′akti) is S′iva as the *Bāṇa Linga*. One distinctive feature of this lotus is that its filaments are tinged with the rays of the sun. The *Anāhata* is described as the great Cakra in the heart of all; *Oṁkāra* is here.

This Lotus is to be distinguished from the Heart Lotus of eight petals which is situate below it. That is not a cakra but a lotus—turned upwards—*Ānanda Kāṇḍa* in which one meditates upon the *Iṣṭa Devatā* in *mānasa pūja*, mental worship.

VIS′UDDHA

Then there is at the spinal centre in the region at the base of the throat, the *Viśuddha Cakra.* It is called thus for the Jīva has attained purity (*viśuddha*) by the sight of the Hamsa. It is also known as the *Bhārati Sthāna* (Home of the Deity of Speech) for it governs the power of expression. It is a lotus of sixteen petals in smoky purple with the vowels, *aṁ*, *āṁ*, *iṁ*, *īṁ*, *uṁ*, *ūṁ*, *ṛṁ*, *ṛṁ*, *lriṁ*, *lrīṁ*, *eṁ*, *aiṁ*, *oṁ*, *ouṁ*, *aṁ*, *aḥ*, in crimson. The governing Tattva is Ether or *Ākāśa*, its colour white and form circular. Its Bīja is *Haṁ*, mounted on a white elephant. Here is *Sadā-Siva* in his form of *Ardhanāriśvara*, *i.e.*, inseparably united with Girija or Gauri, with half the body white and the other half in gold; so also here dwells S′ākini, the S′akti, whose form is light. It is here that the Jñānin becomes *trikāla-darśi*, seer of the three forms of Time.

The author records that above this *Viśuddha Cakra* there is, at the root of the palate, a minor Cakra, *Lālana* or *Kāli Cakra*—a red lotus with twelve petals.

ĀJÑĀ

Still higher up is the *Ājñā Cākra*; it is called as such because here is received from above the command, *ājñā*, of the Guru, who is none else than the Lord S′iva. It is located between the two eye-brows. This lotus has two petals, white in colour, on which are white letters *haṁ* and *kṣaṁ*.[1] The Tattva of this Centre is Manas, or to be exact, this centre is the seat of the subtle Tattvas of Mahat and Prakṛiti. The Bīja is Praṇava, Om. In this bright form of Praṇava shines the *antar-ātmā*, the inner Atmā, lustrous like a flame—and in its light is visible all that is between the *Mūlādhāra* and the *Brahmarandhra*. The deities are Parama S'iva (in the form of Hamsa) and the white Hākinī S'akti.

Here in the inverted triangle, *yoni*, within the pericarp of the lotus, is S'iva as the *Ītara Liñga*.[2]

Above this Cakra are two minor ones:

(1) *Manas Cakra*—lotus of six petals, the seat of "sensations of hearing, touch, sight, smell, taste, and centrally initiated sensations in dream and hallucination".[3]

(2) *Soma Cakra*—lotus of sixteen petals, which are also known as sixteen *kalās* which are so many *vṛttis*.[4]

Above is the region of the Causal Body. "Above this this last Cakra is 'the house without support' (*nirālamba purī*), where yogis see the radiant Īśvara. Above this is the *praṇava* shining like a flame, and above *praṇava* the white crescent

[1] Thus the petals of all the six lotuses total up to fifty and the letters likewise are fifty.

[2] Thus it is seen that there are three Lingas, *Svayambū*, *Bāṇa* and *Ītara* in the three Cakras, Mūlādhāra, Anāhata, and the Ajñā respectively. Here are the three *Granthis* or Knots where the Māyā S'akti is particularly concentrated. The Granthis are the apexes, converging points of the Tattvas regnant in their region. Each region is named after the Deity presiding over it. The region between the Mūlādhāra and the Svādhiṣṭhāna is known as the domain of Fire (*Agni-Khaṇḍa*), with the Brahma Granti above it; between the Manipūra and the Anāhata it is the domain of Sun (*Sūrya-Khaṇḍa*) with the Viṣṇu Granthi above; between the Viśuddha and the Ājñā it is the domain of Moon (*Candra-Khaṇḍa*) with the Rudra Granthi above it. These are the famous Granthis that have to be loosened and undone for yogic liberation to be possible.

[3] *Sabdā -jñāna*, *sparśa-jñāna*, *rūpa-jñāna*, *āghrāṇopa-abdhi*, *rasopabhoga* and *svapna*, with their opposites.

[4] *Kṛpā* (mercy), *mṛḍutvā* (gentleness), *dhairya* (composure), *vāirāgya* (dispassion), *dhṛti* (constancy), *sampat* (prosperity), *hāsya* (cheerfulness), *romānca* (thrill), *vinaya* (humility), *dhyāna* (meditation), *susthiratā* (quietude), *gāmbhirya* (gravity), *udyama* (effort), *akṣobha* (non-agitation), *audārya* (magnanimity) and *ekāgratā* (one-pointedness).

Nāda, and above this last the point, *Bindu*. There is then a White Lotus of twelve petals with its head upwards,[1] over this lotus there is the ocean of nectar (*sudhā sāgara*), the island of gems (*maṇidvīpa*), the altar of gems (*maṇipīṭha*), the forked lightning-like lines, *a*, *ka*, *tha*, and therein *Nāda* and *Bindu*. On Nāda and Bindu, as an altar, there is the *Paramahaṁsa*, and the latter serves as an altar for the feet of the *Guru*; there the *Guru* of all should be meditated. The body of the *Hamsa* on which the feet of the *Guru* rest is *jñāna-māya*, the wings *āgama* and *nigama*, the two feet *śiva* and *śakti*, the beak *praṇava*, the eyes and throat *kāma-kalā*."[2]

Beyond, there is the Sahasrāra, the White Lotus of one thousand petals each of which contains all the Letters of the alphabet, and is the own abode of Para-S'iva. It hangs with head downwards from the Brahmarandhra above all the Cakras. It is the Brahmaloka whence all originates. Whatever exists is first here potentially. This place is *S'iva-Sthāna* for S'aivas, *Parama Puruṣa* for Vaiṣṇavas, *Devi-Sthāna* for S'āktas.

"Above (the end) of the Suṣumnā Nādi is the Lotus of a thousand petals; it is white and has its head downward turned; its filaments are red. The fifty letters of the Alphabet from *A* to *La*, which are also white, go round and round its thousand petals twenty times. On its pericarp is *Hamsa*, and above it is the *Guru* who is *Parama-S'iva* Himself. Above the *Guru* are the *Sūrya* and *Candra-Maṇḍalas*, and above them *Mahāvāyu*. Over the latter is placed Brahmarandhra, and above it *Mahāśankhinī*. In the Maṇḍala of the Moon is the lightning-like triangle within which is the sixteenth *Kalā* of the Moon (*amā kalā*), which is fine as the hundredth part of the lotus-fibre, and of a red colour,

[1] This Lotus forms the subject-matter of the *Pādukā Pāñcaka Stotra*.

[2] *Introduction to Tantra S'āstra*, by Sir John Woodroffe.

with its mouth downward turned. In the lap of this *Kalā* is the *Nirvāṇa Kalā*, subtle like the thousandth part of the end of a hair, also red and with the mouth downward turned.[1] Below the *Nirvāṇa Kalā* is the Fire called *Nibodhikā* which is a form of *Avyakta-nāda*. Above it (Nibodhika), and within Nirvāṇa Kalā, is Para Bindu, which is both S'iva and S'akti. The S'akti of this Para Bindu is the Nirvāṇa S'akti, who is Light (*Tejas*) and exists in the form of *Hamsa* (*Hamsarūpa*), and is subtle like the ten-millionth part of the end of a hair. That *Hamsa* is Jīva. Within the Bindu is the void (*S'ūnya*) which is the *Brahma-pada* (place of Brahman)".[2]

Each of these Cakras is a centre of a Particular Tattva with a *tanmātra* and the Indriyas (sensory and motor organs) connected with it. Thus:

Mūlādhāra	..	Pṛthivī Tattva (Earth) Gandha Tanmātra (Smell) Jñānendriya of smell Karmendriya of feet.
Svādhiṣṭhāna	..	Ap Tattva (Water) Rasa Tanmātra (Taste) Jñānendriya of taste Karmendriya of hands
Maṇipūra	..	Tejas Tattva (Fire) Rūpa Tanmātra (Sight) Jñānendriya of sight Karmendriya of anus
Anāhata	..	Vāyu Tattva (Air) Sparśa Tanmātra (Touch) Jñānendriya of touch Karmendriya of genitals

[1] Read also: "Close to the thousand-petalled lotus is the sixteenth digit of the moon, which is called *āma kalā*, which is pure red and lustrous like lightning, as fine as a fibre of the lotus, hanging downwards, receptacle of the lunar nectar. In it is the crescent *nirvāṇa kalā*, luminous as the Sun, and finer than the thousandth part of hair. This is the Iṣṭa Devata of all. Near *nirvāṇa kalā* is *parama nirvāṇa śakti*, infinitely subtle, lustrous as the Sun, creatrix of *tattva jñāna*. Above it are *Bindu* and *Visarga-śakti*, root and abode of all bliss." (*Introduction to Tantra S'āstra*),

[2] *The Serpent Power*.

Viśuddha	..	Ākāśa Tattva S'abda Tanmātra Jñānendriya of hearing Karmendriya of mouth
Ājñā	..	Subtle Tattvas of Mind Prakṛti

Identifications have been attempted between these Cakras and some of the plexuses in the body. But they are misleading; for the plexuses belong to the gross physical body while the Cakras are subtle vital centres of consciousness. The Cakras are locii—special centres—of operation of the Tattvas which are the self-formulations of the S'akti; they influence, vitalise and control corresponding regions of the body, and the organs, nerves, plexuses, etc., situated in them. In fact it is these subtle concentrations of Consciousness-Power which develop out of themselves, and keep in being, their gross embodiments taking shape into the physical body.

Each of the Cakras has a Deity, a particular form of Consciousness—presiding over it. This form or aspect of Consciousness, the *Devatā*, governs and informs the bodily region around it.[1] And each Deity has its own abode, *Loka*. Thus:

CAKRA	DEITY	LOKA
Mūlādhāra	Brahmā	Bhūrloka
Svādhiṣṭhāna	Rudra	Bhuvarloka
Maṇipūra	Viṣṇu	Svarloka
Anāhata	Īśvara	Janaloka
Viśuddha	Sadāśiva	Tapaloka
Ājñā	S'ambhu	Maharloka

The Sahasrāra, above the six centres, is the place of Parama S'iva whose abode is Satyaloka.

The six Tattvas centred in the six Cakras are, it must be noted, the subtle forms of the respective Devatās. Out of these Tattvas are formed both the gross human body and

[1] Apart from the different regions of the body, the organism as a whole has a distinct consciousness, the Jīva.

the universe—the macrocosm. Hence the Cakras are "the divine subtle centres of the corresponding physical and psychical sheaths".

"The Supreme, therefore, descends through its manifestations from the subtle to the gross as the six Devas and S'aktis in their six abodes in the world-axis, and as the six centres in the body-axis or spinal column. The special operation of each of the Tattvas is located at its individual centre in the microcosm. But, not-withstanding all such subtle and gross transformations of and by Kula Kuṇḍalinī, She ever remains in Her Brahman or Svarūpa aspect the One, Sat, Cit, and Ānanda, as is realised by the Yogī when drawing the Devī from Her world abode in the earth centre (*mūlādhāra*) he unites Her with Para-S'iva in the Sahasrāra in that blissful union which is the Supreme Love (Ānanda)."[1]

Regarding the *letters* which are on the petals of the Lotus it goes without saying that they are not the gross letters seen by the common eye. In a remarkably brilliant exposition, the author explains :

"Each object of perception, whether gross or subtle, has an aspect which corresponds to each of the senses. It is for this reason that the Tantra correlates sound, form and colour. Sound produces form, and form is associated with colour. Kuṇḍalī is a form of the Supreme S'akti who maintains all breathing creatures; She is the source from which all sound or energy, whether as ideas or speech, manifests. That sound or Mātṛkā when uttered in human speech assumes the form of letters and prose and verse, which is made of their combinations. And sound (S'abdā) has its meaning—that is, the objects denoted by the ideas which are expressed by sound or words. By the impulse of Icchā śakti acting through the Prāṇa Vāyu (vital force)

[1] *The Serpent Power.*

of the Ātma is produced in the Mūlādhāra the sound power called Parā, which in its ascending movement through other Cakras takes on other characteristics and names (Paśyantī and Madhyamā), and when uttered by the mouth appears as Vaikhari in the form of the spoken letters which are the gross aspect of the sound in the Cakras themselves. Letters when spoken are, then, the manifested aspect in gross speech of the subtle energy of the S'abda-brahman as Kuṇḍalī. The same energy which produces these letters manifesting as Mantras produces the gross universe. In the Cakras is subtle S'abda in its states as Parā, Paśyantī, or Madhyamā-S'akti, which when translated to the vocal organ assumes the audible sound form (*dhvani*) which is any particular letter. Particular forms of energy of Kuṇḍalī are said to be resident at particular Cakras, all such energies existing in magnified form in the Sahasrāra. Each manifested letter is a Mantra, and a Mantra is the body of a Devatā. There are therefore as many Devatās in a Cakra as there are petals which are surrounding (*Āvaraṇa*) Devatās or S'aktis of the Devatā of the Cakra and the subtle element of which He is the presiding Consciousness. Thus, Brahmā is the presiding Consciousness of the Mūlādhāra lotus, indicated by the Bindu of the Bīja La (*Laṁ*), which is the body of the earth Devatā; and round and associated with these are subtle forms of the Mantras, which constitute the petals and the bodies of associated energies. The whole human body is in fact a Mantra, and is composed of Mantras. These sound powers vitalize, regulate, and control the corresponding gross manifestations in the regions surrounding them."[1]

[1] *The Serpent Power.*

CHAPTER FIVE

YOGA

EVERY Jīva is in essence the Paramātma; each individual self is God. But this identity is veiled by Māyā, *Avidyā*—Ignorance, and the being appears to be separate from God. The process by which this sense of separativity is eliminated and the Jīvātma regains his oneness with the Paramātma is Yoga.

As the sense of separateness is caused by Ignorance, *Avidyā*, the realisation of identity is brought about by *Vidyā* or *Jñāna*. This *Jñāna* is of two kinds:

(1) *Svarūpa Jñāna*, the knowledge of the utmost Pure Consciousness,

(2) *Kriyā Jñāna*, the means to gain the former. It consists of the mental process of discrimination of what is Brahman and what is not and the concentration of the mind on what is Brahman until, by a progressive absorption into Brahman, one loses oneself in it. This gradual liberation is called the *Kramamukti* which is ultimately perfected into *Jīvanmukti*, liberation even while in the body, culminating into the supreme Liberation, *parama-mukti*, after death.

But man is not the mind alone. He has emotions; he has a life-dynamism; he has a body. So there are processes (yogas) which are associated with them also, *e.g.*, means of devotion and worship, Bhakti Yoga, Mantra Yoga; mental control and subtilisation of life-energy, *prāṇa*, Rāja Yoga; purification and perfection of the physical body, Hatha Yoga. The main principle underlying all these processes is that the ceaseless activities of the mental, emotive and vital faculties, *citta*, *vṛtti*, and *prāṇa*, which always cover up, *āvaraṇa*, screen the true nature of one's consciousness, Cit, must be stayed and controlled. It is only when this is effectively done and all is still, that there arises the perception of true Cit as one's own nature; this state, the natural state of the self, is called *samādhi*—the condition in which the equality, the oneness of Jīvātma and Paramātmā is realised.

Though these several forms of Yoga have one aim—the realisation of the Brahman or Pure Consciousness as one's real nature, their means differ. Yet there is an underlying preparatory discipline common to all; it is the eight-limbed, *aṣṭānga*, discipline for the purification and equipment for the deeper practice of Yoga. It consists of:

(1) *Yama*, restraint. It is tenfold: abstinence from injury, *ahimsā;* truthfulness, *satyam;* non-covetousness, *asteyam;* continence, *brahmacarya;* forbearance, *kṣamā;* fortitude, *dhṛti;* kindliness, *dayā;* simplicity, *ārjavam;* moderation in diet, *mitāhāra;* and purity of mind and body, *śaucam.*

(2) *Niyama*, observance, also tenfold. Austerities for purificatory purposes, *tapaḥ;* contentment, *santoṣa;* belief in the Veda, *āstikyam;* charity, *dānam;* worship of God, *pūjanam;* hearing of the authentic word, *śravaṇam;* shame at wrong action, *hṛī;* mind habitually inclined to higher knowledge and practice prescribed in the S'āstra, *mati;* recitation of Mantra, *japa;* sacrifice, *hutam*, or religious observances, *vrata.*

(3) *Āsana*, posture of the body which is most favourable for the practice of Yoga, by promoting solidity in the physical frame and free circulation of energy in the system. Each one has to find which posture is the most steady and pleasant to him. The perfect *āsana* is one in which the spine and the head are erect, there is no movement of the body and the mind falls into a state of equilibrium.[1] Certain Yogas like

[1] Among the most common and convenient are the *Mukta-padma-āsana* and

the Haṭha·Yoga have specialised in this subject and evolved a number of intricate Āsanas yielding amazing results.

(4) *Prāṇāyāma*—lengthening (*āyama*) of *Prāṇa*, life-breath, by a process of the regulation and development of the life-breath. The inhaling and exhaling of air is controlled with a view to make the vital airs equable and produce a state favourable for mental concentration.

(5) *Pratyāhāra*, restraint of the senses from their customary pursuits. They are reined in and subjected to the conscious rule of the mind. The mind is withdrawn from the sense-objects and steadied.

These are the five exterior (*bahiranga*) methods followed by the three interior (*antaranga*) which are:

(6) *Dhāraṇa*, concentration and fixing, the 'holding of the mind', *citta*, on a particular object of thought.

(7) *Dhyāna*, continued dwelling upon or contemplation of the object so held (in *dhāraṇa*). The consciousness is occupied by the thought of one object; either an object with form, *saguṇa*, or without form, *nirguṇa*. In the former there is *dhyāna* of a *mūrti;* in the latter, the self is the object, leading ultimately to a consciousness of the object alone.

(8) *Samādhi.* This state when complete is the state of *Para-Samvit*, Pure Consciousness. There are two degrees of the samādhi; the first, *savikalpa*, when the mind increasingly becomes one with the subject of its contemplation—a condition of trance or ecstasy; the second, *nirvikalpa*, when it is completely identified with and lost in it.

In the Vedāntic classification, the Savikalpa Samādhi

---

the *Baddha-Padma asana*: In the former the right foot is first placed on the left thigh and the left on the right thigh; hands crossed and placed similarly on the thighs; with the chin on the breast the gaze is fixed on the tip of the nose. In the *baddha-padma*, the position of the feet is the same; but the hands are passed behind the back and the right hand is made to hold the right toe and the left hand the left toe. This increases the pressure on the Mūlādhāra and the nerves are toned up as the body tightens.

(known as the *Samprajñāta*) is further seen in three stages: (1) *Ṛtambharā*, where the knower is still separate from the known and the movement of mind is filled with *saccidānanda.* (2) *Prajñālokā*, where all covering, *āvaraṇa*, ceases and there is *Brahma-Jñāna*. (3) *Praśāntavāhitā* wherein all modification, *vṛtti*, ceases and the self is nothing but pure Brahman. It is a state of utmost peace. This is the door to Nirvikalpa Samādhi.

"Thus by Yama, Niyama, Āsana, the body is controlled; by these and Prāṇāyāma the Prāṇa is controlled; by these and Pratyāhāra the senses (Indriyas) are brought under subjection. Then through the operation of Dhāraṇā, Dhyānā and the lesser Samādhi (Savikalpa or Samprajñāta) the modifications (*vṛtti*) of the Manas cease and Buddhi alone functions. By the further and long practice of dispassion or indifference to both joy and sorrow (*vairāgya*) Buddhi itself becomes *Laya*, and the Yogi attains the true unmodified state of the Ātma, in which the Jīva who is then pure Buddhi is merged in Prakṛti and the Brahman, as salt in the waters of ocean and as camphor in the flame."[1]

Coming to the specialities of some of the more important Yogas in so far as they shed helpful light on the subject of Kuṇḍalinī Yoga, we first take up the Mantra Yoga as it is the simplest.

MANTRA YOGA

The mind is constantly modifying itself (*vṛtti*) in the form of the objects it perceives; it busies itself with things in the spirit or feeling, *bhāva*, which they induce in it. The object of the Mantra Yoga is to place a form—*Nāma-rūpa*, which produces a pure *bhāva*, as the object of contemplation

[1] *The Serpent Power.*

and adoration before the mind; the forms are images, *mūrti*, emblems, *liṇga*, *śāligrāma*, pictures, *citra*, mural markings, *bhitti rekhā*, diagrams, *maṇḍala* and *yantra*. This is called *saguṇa dhyāna*.[1] This is accompanied by *Japa*, repetition of a prescribed mantra, audibly or inaudibly. The Mantra is the sound-equivalent (body) of a particular Devata, and its intonation evokes the Deity embodied in it. Fixation of the gaze in particular ways, *mudrā*, and touching of the body in certain parts, *nyāsa*, are enjoined during the Japa.

The eight limbs described earlier enter into this discipline as in the other yogas. This practice of Japa and meditation in worship leads to a state of Samādhi which is here called the *Mahā-bhāva*. We may note in passing that the object of this Yoga is the attainment of the formless One by Jñāna. The *saguṇa dhyāna* is a process that leads to it; it is the least complicated method which does not call for any special development in the sādhaka. "The Deva of the unawakened is in Images; of the *vipras* in Fire; of the wise in the Heart. The Deva of those who know the Ātma is everywhere." (*Kulārṇava Tantra*, IX. 44).

HAṬHA YOGA

Haṭha is a compound of the syllable *Ha* which stands for 'Sun' and *Ṭha* for 'Moon', the Sun being the *Prāṇa-vāyu* and the Moon *Apāna-vāyu*. The Prāṇa (in the heart) and the Apāna (in the Mūlādhāra) constantly draw each other and it is this mutual disagreement that prevents them from leaving the body, thus, maintaining a continuous life-activity.

[1] It is also called *sthūla dhyāna*, since the form of the Deity contemplated is *sthūla*, with limbs, etc. The Dhyāna in which the form of the Mūrti is *sūkṣma*, subtle, the *mantra*, is *sūkṣma dhyāna*. There is yet a third, still subtler form, the supreme, *para* form of the Deity, *Vāsana* which is its own form.

To still this activity the two currents are to be regulated into agreement. Their union and the process leading to it is *Prāṇāyāma*. The Prāṇa in the individual body is part of the Universal Prāṇa—the Great Breath; Haṭha Yoga seeks to harmonise the individual breath with the Cosmic Breath. This results in the increase of strength and health and the steadiness of mind and concentration.

Prāṇāyāma—the regulation and the processing of the life-breath, plays the chief part in this yoga for the achievement of Mokṣa. The stress here being on Prāṇa as the determinant of the *vṛttis* of Manas, all effort is directed towards the union of *Ha* and *Ṭha* in the Suṣumnā and their advance upwards[1] through the several Cakras to the Brahmarandhra for the attainment of Samādhi. Side by side, there are a number of physical practices developed in this yoga for the control and purification of the body which facilitates Prāṇāyāma. It is not necessary here to go into these details. We may only note they are: cleansing, *śodhana*[2]; acquiring firmness, *dṛḍhatā*, by āsanas; fortitude, *sthiratā*, by mudrās, postures of the body; steadiness of mind, *dhairya*, by restraint of sense; lightness, *lāghava*, by prāṇāyāma; realisation, *pratyakṣa*, by meditation, dhyāna; and detachment, *nirliptatva* through Samādhi[3] (known here as the *Mahā-bodha* Samādhi) which culminates in Mukti, liberation.

1 Which is rendered possible by the stirring and movement of Kuṇḍalinī awakened in the process—as will be described in the next chapter.

2 By six processes, *ṣaṭ-karma: dhauti*, washing of the stomach by a piece of cloth, *vasti*, cleaning of the colon by drawing in water, *nauli* or *lauliki*, rolling of intestines from side to side, *kapālabhāti* (breathing bellow-like), *neti* (cleaning of nostrils by strings), and *trāṭaka* (one-pointed gaze).

3 "Samādhī considered as a process is intense mental concentration, with freedom from all *saṁkalpa*, and attachment to the world, and all sense of 'mineness' or self-interest (*mamatā*). Considered as the result of such process it is the union of Jīva with Paramātma" (*Introduction to Tantra S'āstra*).

RĀJA YOGA

In this yoga the main emphasis is laid on the mental faculties. It employs the methods of *āsana* and *prāṇāyāma*, but mainly for the purpose of marshalling and canalising the life-energies in such a manner as to eliminate obstruction of tamas and ignorance in the system and quiet the activity of the mind. Here the aim is Nirvikalpa Samādhi which is higher than the Savikalpa attainable in the other yogas hitherto considered. In fact the Savikalpa prepares the way for the Nirvikalpa Samādhi. The *Vairāgya*, detachment, that characterises this state of consciousness is the highest type, *Para.*[1] The mind is decisively turned away from the objects of the world—a complete *pratyāhāra*—and cannot be turned back. The mind is rigorously trained to discriminate the Real from the unreal, the Infinite from the finite, the Soul from the non-soul, by its own reasoning purified in the fire of *Vairāgya*, and with the aid of the authentic teaching of the *S'āstra*. It has to realise that the Reality is self-existent, is conscious and is blissful. By constant *vicāra* and *dhāraṇā* and *dhyāna*, the mind passes through the Savikalpa Samādhi into the state of Nirvikalpa Samādhi and loses itself in the state of the Pure Self—the final Liberation even while being in the body—*Jivanmukti*.

Next we come to the *Laya* or the *Kuṇḍalinī* Yoga.

[1] As distinguished from the Vairāgya of *mṛdu* type which is inconstant and weak, the *madhyama* where there is desire in the face of opportunity but no yearning in its absence, the *adhimātra* where pleasures of the world become a source of misery.

CHAPTER SIX

KUṆḌALINĪ YOGA

THE Twin principles of Creation, Consciousness in itself and Consciousness as Power, S′iva and S′akti in the terminology of the Tāntric system, are there reproduced in each form of the universe. In the human body the Pure Consciousness, S′iva, is stationed in its highest cerebral centre, the *Sahasrāra*, and the Consciousness-Power, the Prakṛti-S′akti, is located in the lowest centre, the *Mūlādhāra*. Normally this S′akti is latent and it is only through its secondary manifestations *e.g.* the several forms of *Vāyu Prāna*, that the organism is sustained and kept going. To awaken this 'sleeping' Power, control and unite it with its Master Consciousness at the summit, to merge the power of the Body into the power of the Soul is the object of this Yoga. This union results in an ecstatic samādhi in which the whole system is flooded by Ānanda and the individual consciousness gets one with the supreme Consciousness—Jīva becomes one with S′iva.

The S′akti, the fundamental Power which bases and governs each human organism is called the *Kula-Kuṇḍalī*; it is imaged as lying coiled up (*Kuṇḍalī*). It is the *Parā S′akti* in the body of which all other forces and powers are manifestations. She is also known as *Kutilāngī*, the crooked one, *Bhujangī*, serpent, *Īśvarī*, etc. The Serpent Power lies coiled up (3½ times) in the Mūlādhāra, with its mouth closing the entrance to the Suṣumnā, the *Brahmadvāra*, door to Brahman. The Kuṇḍalinī is just above the root of the Nādis, called the *Kanda* (which is generally said to be two fingers above the anus and two fingers below the generative organs). The

Kula Kuṇḍalinī is also the *S'abda Brahman*—Nāda S'akti in the body and all mantras are Her formulations. She is the source of all Speech. So too are the six centres the manifestations of this creative power. Prāṇa is a particular manifestation of this Kuṇḍalinī S'akti and the process of awakening her begins with a concentrated stress on Prāṇa. The exact process is to be learnt from the Guru. Yet, briefly described, without entering into the deeper technicalities of it, the sādhana proceeds as follows. It is of course presumed that the practicant has equipped himself with sufficient training in the preparatory discipline of the *Aṣṭānga*, Yama, Niyama, etc.

The sādhaka sits in a prescribed *āsana* and steadies the mind by concentrating between the eye-brows. Air is inhaled and retained; the upper part of the body is contracted and the *prāṇa* (upward breath) is checked. The air thus prevented from going upward tends to rush downward; this escape of *vāyu* as *apāna* is also checked by appropriate contraction of the lower parts. The *vāyu* thus collected is directed towards the Mūlādhāra centre and the mind and will are concentrated upon it with the result that due to the frictional pressure of Prāṇa and Apāna held tight together, intense heat is generated and this again arouses the sleeping serpent, *Kuṇḍalinī*, which when so activated is drawn upwards. By mental concentration with the aid of *mantra*, the *jīvātma* which is of the shape of a flame is brought down from the heart to the Mūlādhāra and, so to say, united and moved along with the awakened S'akti. As its coils are loosened, the aperture to the door of Brahman, *Brahmadvāra*, at the mouth of the Suṣumnā, is opened and through the Citrini Nādi within, the Kuṇḍalinī is led upwards.[1]

[1] "The Yogi should sit in the proper posture and place his two hands with palms upwards in his lap and steady his mind (citta) by the *khecari mudrā*. He should next fill the interior of his body with air and hold it in by *kumbhaka*, and contract

"The Āsanas, Kumbhakas, Bandhas, and Mudras, are used to rouse the Kuṇḍalinī, so that the Prāṇa withdrawn from Iḍā and Pingalā may by the power of its S'akti, after entry into the Suṣumnā or void (*śūnya*), go upwards towards the Brahmarandhra. The Yogi is then said to be free of the active karma, and attain the natural state. The object, then, is to devitalise the rest of the body getting the Prāṇa from Iḍā and Pingalā into Suṣumnā, . . . and then to make it ascend through the lotuses which 'bloom' on its approach. The body on each side of the spinal column is devitalised and the whole current of Prāṇa thrown into that column."[2]

"The principle of all the methods to attain Samādhi is to get the Prāṇa out of Iḍā and Pingalā. When this is achieved these Nādīs become 'dead', because vitality has gone out of them. The Prāṇa then enters the Suṣumnā and, after piercing by the aid of Kuṇḍalinī the six Cakras in the Suṣumnā, becomes Laya or absorbed in the Sahasrāra. The means to this end, when operating from the Mūlādhāra, seem to vary in detail, but embody a common principle, namely, the forcing of Prāṇa downward and Apāna upwards, (that is, the reverse of their natural directions) by the *Jālandhara* and *Mūlabandha*, or otherwise, when by their union the internal fire is increased. The position seems to be thus similar to a hollow tube in which a piston is working at both ends without escape of the central air, which thus become heated. Then the Serpent Force, Kuṇḍalinī, aroused by the heat thus

---

the heart. By so doing the escape of the upward breath is stopped. Then, when he feels that the air within him from the belly to the throat is tending downward through the channels in the Nādis, he should contract the anus and stop the downward air (*āpāna*); then again having raised the air, let him give the *Kāma-vāyu* within the triangle in the pericarp of the Mūlādhāra Lotus a turn from the left to the right (*vāmavartena*); by so doing the fire of *Kāma* there is kindled, and Kuṇḍalinī gets heated (excited) thereby: He should then pierce the mouth of the Svāyambhūlinga, and through its aperture with the aid of the 'Hum' Bīja, lead Her who desires union with Parama-Sīva within the mouth of the Citrinī Nādi." *The Serpent Power.*

[2] *The Serpent Power.*

generated, is aroused from her potential state called 'sleep' in which she lies curled up. She then hisses and straightens Herself, and enters the Brahmadvāra, or enters into the Suṣumnā, when by further repeated efforts the Cakras in the Suṣumnā are pierced. This is a gradual process which is accompanied by special difficulties at the three knots (Granthis) where Māyā S′akti is powerful, particularly the abdominal knot, the piercing of which may, it is admitted, involve considerable pain, physical disorder, and even disease."[1]

As the S′akti darts upward and forces its way[2] it strikes against each of the lotuses which then bloom upwards.[3] This is the famous *Cakra Bheda;* the piercing of the Centres. Advancing from Centre to Centre, the S′akti swallows up the Tattvas that are embodied or concentrated in them. Each Tattva is absorbed in the next subtler Tattva (which is its immediate cause) and all are dissolved into the Cid-Ātma.

[1] *The Serpent Power.*

[2] There is a difference of opinion and a lively controversy in which Sir John Woodroffe participates, as to whether it is the Kuṇḍalinī S′akti itself that goes upwards or it is only an *eject* of it that is thrown up. The latter position is taken up by the well-known authority on Tantra S′āstra, S′rī Pramatha Natha Mukhyopadhyaya, now Swāmi Pratyāgātmānanda.

[3] During the preparation of this manuscript, an interesting book has come into our hands—*Light on the Path of Self-Realization* (Publ. by N. V. Gunaji, Thalakwadi, Belgaum, 1941). It contains, among other things, recorded statements of their experiences in S′adhana by a group of practitioners of yoga. A few excerpts from one of them will be found apposite by way of practical illustration of some of the truths presented in this exposition:

"....Then suddenly a light began to be seen, which day by day increased so that sunshine appeared to be spreading and I began to feel the heat......Then there was a change in the nature of the light which appeared as cool as moonlight and a sensation of joy and calmness was experienced. Some days later, black stones appeared near the heart and flames of fire were seen coming out of them. Some days later a stalk came up from the flames and from it there appeared to be hanging with its mouth downwards something like the flower of the plantain tree. Some days later the flower instead of hanging down turned its face upwards. Mahārāja (Guru) said: 'This is the lotus near the heart. You will see it distinctly in a few days and its petals will be opened.' The flames then ceased to come out and below

"As Kuṇḍalinī united with the subtle Jīvātma passes through each of these lotuses, She absorbs into Herself the regnant Tattvas of each of these centres, and all that has been above described to be in them. As the ascent is made, each of the grosser Tattvas enters into the Laya state, and is replaced by the energy of the Kuṇḍalinī, which after the passage of the *Viśuddha-Cakra* replaces them all. The senses which operate in association with these grosser Tattvas are merged in Her, who then absorbs into Herself the subtle Tattvas of the Ājñā. Kuṇḍalinī Herself takes on a different aspect as She ascends the three planes, and unites with each of the Lingas in that form of Hers which is appropriate to such union. For whereas in the Mūlādhāra She is the S'akti of all in their gross or physical manifested state (*Virāṭ*), at the stage of Ājñā, She is the S'akti of the mental and psychic or subtle body (*Hiraṇya-garbha*), and in the region of the Sahasrāra She is the S'akti of the 'spiritual' plane (*Īśvara*), which though itself in its S'iva aspect is undifferentiated, contains in its Power aspect all lower planes in a concealed potential state. . . .

---

the stalk appeared something like water. Then the petals began one by one to open, some up and some down, and a red lotus similar to that which is generally drawn below the picture of the goddess, came in view.

"After some days black spots appeared on the petals in which spots, some days later there appeared shapes of letters. I asked M. whether there were actual letters in the spots. He replied that they were the seeds of that lotus and that he would later on take me to the navel lotus. . . .

"Then I proceeded towards the navel lotus. There first appeared terrible flames of fire. Some days later the navel lotus appeared. It was similar to the lotus of the heart but the petals were slightly different. Many days later the form of Śeṣasāyi (Viṣṇu sleeping on the snake) appeared but it was indistinct. From the navel of Viṣṇu issued forth a lotus plant and Brahmadeva appeared to be sitting on the flower. . . .

"Then once M. said: 'I shall show you the Kuṇḍalinī today. In Yoga practice the Kuṇḍalinī is the most important spot; you sit now and go below Ganapati'. I did so and after some time, I saw a triangular pit near the hip-bone, much below Ganapati. Furious flames of fire were darting out of it. I felt a burning sensation in various parts of the body and my whole body was perspiring. I had previously

"The upward movement is from the gross to the more subtle, and the order of dissolution of the Tattvas is as follows: Pṛthivī with the Indriyas (smell and feet), the latter of which have Pṛthivī (the earth as ground) as their support, is dissolved into Gandha-Tattva, or Tanmātra of smell, which is in the Mūlādhāra: Gandha-Tattva is then taken to Svādhiṣṭhāna, and it, Ap, and its connected Indriyas (taste and hands), are dissolved in Rasa (Taste) Tanmātra; the latter is taken to the Maṇipūra and there Rasa-Tattva, Tejas, and its connected Indriyas (sight and anus), are dissolved into Rūpa (sight) Tanmātra; then the latter is taken into the Anāhata, and it, Vāyu, and the connected Indriyas (touch and penis), are dissolved in Sparśa (Touch) Tanmātra; the latter is taken to the Viśuddha, and there it, Ākāśa, and associated Indriyās (hearing and mouth) are dissolved in the S′abda (sound) Tanmātra; the latter is then taken to the Ājñā, and, there and beyond it, Manas is dissolved in Mahat, Mahat in Sūkṣma Prakṛti, and the latter is united with Para Bindu in the Sahasrāra. In the case of the latter merger there are various stages. . . .as of *Nāda*

seen flames twice or thrice but they were not so extremely hot as these. Every day this sight continued to appear for some days. Then the flames disappeared and I could clearly make out the triangular pit. Two small pipes close to each other appeared to come out of the pit and go upwards. Between the two pipes there appeared a hollow space of the same size as that of the pipes. Below the pipes there appeared a black snake which had coiled itself round the pipes. I asked M. about this to which he replied, 'The two small pipes are the two nerves Iḍā and Pingalā and the hollow space in the middle is the Suṣumnā. These three are the main nerves. When we breathe through the nose, we breathe through these nerves. The snake which you saw below the pipes is the Kuṇḍalinī. It is always asleep in the ordinary human body. Its mouth is near the opening of the belly and it always swallows nectar. When the Kuṇḍalinī awakes, a man becomes a Yogi. To awaken it a man has to proceed very carefully along the path of Yoga observing many restrictions. If it is awakened and its mouth is not turned upwards, a man will not live. Hence the person who awakens it must have great power. As the Kuṇḍalinī proceeds upwards through the Suṣumnā nerve, the man gets more and more powers. I shall tell about this in detail later on. Let us now go to the two-petalled lotus.'

"M. told me that now I must direct my eye-sight upwards *i.e.*, I must fix it between into *Nādānta* into *Vyāpikā*, *Vyāpikā* into *Samani*, *Samani* into *Unmanī*, and the latter into *Viṣṇu-vakira* or *Puṁ-bindu*, which is also *Paramaśiva*. When all the letters have been thus dissolved, all the six Cakras are dissolved as the petals of the lotuses bear the letters.

"On this upward movement, Brahmā, Sāvitrī, Dākinī, the Devas, Mātṛkās, and Vṛttis, of the Mūlādhāra, are absorbed in Kuṇḍalinī, as is also the Mahīmaṇḍala, or Pṛthivī, and the Pṛthivī-Bīja 'Lam' into which it passes. For these Bījas, or sound powers, express the subtle Mantra aspect of that which is dissolved in them. Thus 'earth' springs from and is dissolved in its seed (Bīja), which is that particular aspect of the creative consciousness, which propelled it. The uttered mantra (*Vaikharī śabda*) or 'Lam' is the expression in gross sound of that.

---

the tip of the nose and centre between the eye-brows. This practice then was commenced from that day. . . . After some days' practice I began to see the two-petalled lotus. When M. asked me to describe it, I said that it had a petal on each side. He said, 'That is the *Dvidal* (Two-petalled lotus). It is the place of the Guru. Whenever we want the Darśan of our Guru, we should fix our mind there. But let us proceed further. After further practice an eye began to be seen above the forehead. I asked M. about this eye. He said that it was the third eye of Śrī Śankar and asked me to proceed further. He added, 'I am just showing these places to you. You must fix your mind at each place and secure it. Without this you will not get the power of that place. The reason why I show you these places is that even if you practise in my absence and your astral body (*i.e.*, mind) goes a little astray, still it would remember this and come back to the proper place. Hence I have shown you all these different paths. Now I am no longer needed. You must continue the study and attain the goal of human life. There will be absolutely no danger to you. Now there is only one place to be shown and that is the Sahasradala (the thousand petalled lotus). We shall proceed to that place from tomorrow'.

"Practice was continued from next day. One or two places were seen but not distinctly and hence I cannot describe them. Still I could distinguish Om among them.

"After leaving Om as I proceeded further, something like a majestic temple appeared at a great distance. I think that the thousand-petalled lotus was situated in the interior of that temple as it had innumerable petals difficult to be counted. It was so dazzlingly brilliant that I could not even look at it, by the internal sight. It was therefore, almost impossible for a novice like me to approach it. . . . The light there was of a bluish colour and extremely lustrous."

"When the Devī leaves the Mūlādhāra, that lotus, which by reason of the awakening of Kuṇḍalinī, and the vivifying intensity of the Prāṇik current had opened and turned its flower upwards, again closes and hangs its head downwards. As Kuṇḍalinī reaches the Svādhiṣṭhāna, that lotus opens out and lifts its flower upwards. Upon Her entrance, Viṣṇu, Lakṣmī, Sarasvati, Rākinī, Mātṛkās and Vṛtti, Vaikuṇṭha-dhāma, Goloka, and the Deva and Devī residing therein, are dissolved in the body of the Kuṇḍalinī. The Pṛthivī or earth Bīja 'Lam' is dissolved in the Tattva water, and water converted into its Bīja 'Vam' remains in the body of Kuṇḍalinī. When the Devī reaches the Maṇipūra Cakra or Brahma-granthi, all that is in that Cakra merges in Her. The Varuṇa-Bīja 'Vam' is dissolved in fire, which remains in Her body as the Bīja 'Ram'. The S'akti next reaches the Anāhata Cakra, which is known as the Knot of Viṣṇu (Viṣṇu-granthi), where also all which is therein is merged in Her. The Bīja of Fire 'Ram' is sublimed in air, and air converted into its Bīja 'Yam' is absorbed in Kuṇḍalinī. She then ascends to the abode of Bhāratī or Sarasvati, Viśuddha Cakra. Upon Her entrance, Ardha-nārīśvara S'iva, S'ākini, the 16 vowels, Mantra, etc., are dissolved in Her. The Bīja of Air 'Yam' is dissolved in ether, which, itself being transformed into the Bīja 'Ham', is merged in the body of Kuṇḍalinī. Piercing the concealed Lalanā Cakra, the Devī reaches the Ājñā known as the 'Knot of Rudra' (Rudra-granthi), where Paramaśiva, Siddha-Kālī, the Devas, and all else therein, are dissolved in Her. At length the Bīja of Vyoma (ether) or 'Ham' is absorbed into the subtle Tattvas of the Ājñā, and then into the Devī. After passing through the Rudra-granthi, Kuṇḍalinī is united with Paramaśiva. As She proceeds upwards from the two-petalled lotus, the Nirālambapurī, Praṇava, Nāda, and so forth, are merged in the Devī. She has thus in Her progress upwards absorbed in Herself the twenty-three Tattvas, commencing with the gross elements, and then remaining Herself S'akti as Consciousness, the cause of all S'aktis, unites with Paramaśiva whose nature is one with Hers. . . .

"On their union nectar (*amṛta*) flows, which in ambrosial stream runs from the Brahmarandhra to the Mūlādhāra, flooding the *Kṣudra Brahmāṇḍa*, or microcosm, and satisfying the Devatās of its Cakras. It is then that the sādhaka, forgetful of all in this world, is immersed in ineffable bliss. Refreshment, increased power and enjoyment, follows upon each visit to the Well of Life. . . .

"Kuṇḍalinī having pierced the fourteen 'Knots' (Granthis) —*viz.* three Lingas, six Cakras, and the five S'ivas which they contain, and then Herself drunk of the nectar which issues from Para-S'iva, returns along the path whence She came to Her own abode (Mūlādhāra). As She returns She pours Herself into the Cakras all that She had previously absorbed therefrom. In other words, as Her passage upwards was *Laya-krama*, causing all things in the Cakras to pass into the Laya state (dissolution), so Her return is *Sṛṣti-krama*, as She 'recreates' or makes them manifest. In this manner She again reaches the Mūlādhāra, when all that has been already described to be in the Cakras appears in the positions which they occupied before Her awakening. In fact, the descending Jīvātma makes for himself the idea of that separated multiple and individualised world which passed from him as he ascended to and became one with the Cause. She as Consciousness absorbs what She as conscious Power projected. In short, the return of Kuṇḍalinī is the setting again of the Jīvātma in the phenomenal world of the lowest plane of being after he had been raised therefrom in a state of ecstasis, or Samādhi. The Yogi thus knows (because he experiences) the nature and state of Spirit and its pathway to and from the Māyik and embodied world. In this Yoga there is a gradual process of involution of the gross world with its elements into its Cause. Each gross element (Mahābhūta), together with the subtle element (Tanmātra) from which it proceeds and the connected organ of sense (Indriya), is dissolved into the next above until the last element, ether, with the Tanmātra sound and Manas, are dissolved in Egoism (Ahaṅkāra), of which they are Vikṛtis. Ahaṅkāra is merged in Mahat, the first manifestation of creative ideation, and the latter into Bindu, which is the Supreme Being, Consciousness, and Bliss as the creative Brahman. Kuṇḍalī ascends, the lower limbs become as inert and cold as a corpse; so also does every part of the body when She has passed through and leaves it. This is due to the fact that She as the Power which supports the body as an organic whole is leaving Her centre. On the contrary, the upper part of the head becomes 'lustrous' by which is not meant any external lustre (Prabhā), but brightness, warmth, and animation. When the Yoga is complete, the Yogi sits rigid in the posture selected, and the only trace of warmth to be found in the whole body is at the crown of the head, where the S'akti is united with S'iva."[1]

But the Kuṇḍalinī does not stay in the Sahasrāra for long. There is always a natural tendency to return to its original position. The Yogī has to repeat the process of ascent and descent again and again, strive to retain Her above for longer and longer periods, till the S'akti stays permanently with the Lord,—returning only when so willed (by the Yogī), that is, till the union is complete and the Liberation, Mukti, attains its full form. He is then a Jīvanmukta.

It is to be noted that in this Yoga it is not the faculties of the mind alone that are yoked to the will for liberation

[1] *The Serpent Power.*

as in the Jñāna and allied Yogas where Mukti is sought to be attained by detachment from the world, by mental disciplines like concentration, meditation, etc. the stress being on the capacities and powers of the mental being, the Jñāna S′akti of the seeker. Here the power that effectuates the Sādhana is the Kuṇḍalinī S′akti, the mother of all S′aktis, who, when awakened, herself bestows Jñāna in its amplitude on the individual. Further, the Agency here is a fundamental Power which governs the body, the life and the mind and its aim is not only to unite the Jīva with the S′iva, to release the individual-bound consciousness into the free, illimitable Pure Consciousness, *Mukti*, but equally to bathe the entire being, the body, the mind and the life-energies with the nectar, the ecstasy that flows from such a union, *Bhukti.* The Siddhi is naturally more complete—as not only the mind but the rest of the person also participates in the Joy. This ecstasy is attained in different forms at different centres of the ascent along with their characteristic *siddhis*, supernormal powers, until one arrives at the highest seat, the *Sahasrāra*, which is sheer Bliss-*Kevalānandarūpam*.

APPENDIX

KUṆḌALINĪ YOGA

H. H. Jaya Chamaraja Wadiyar
Maharaja of Mysore

It is a pleasure to welcome Sir John Woodroffe's (Arthur Avalon's) book on *Serpent Power* brought out by Messrs. Ganesh and Co. A unique and very helpful and useful method employed in this new edition is the inclusion of separate indices for the author's verses, citations and words. This thoughtful addition will be of enormous benefit to scholar and savant and ordinary reader alike. The book is well got up, the illustrations are excellent, and we become aware of the fact that Indian printing is second to none, thanks to the labour of love that is bestowed on this book by the printers.

It is not necessary for me to say anything about Sir John Woodroffe, who is already known. Woodroffe has become so much a part of our lives and tradition as one who has re-kindled India's interest in her great Tāntric Sāstras. His service here is inestimable.

One of the main doctrines of Hinduism consists in its worship of S′akti as the ultimate force that governs the world. We find similarly doctrines emphasising the greatness of S′iva or Viṣṇu. Each of these has a theology of its own as well as different forms by which worship is conducted. Of these, Tantra is that which deals with S′āktism in particular, containing philosophical treatises, theology, Yogic practices, ritual, dialectic, etc.

Kuṇḍalini Yoga is one of the most important of the S′akti

Tantras. It is spoken of in the Yoga Upaniṣads, in the Āgamas, and other esoteric works. The S'akti known as Kuṇḍalinī is one which is found within everyone. Kuṇḍalinī Yoga is the method by which that which is coiled, at the root-centre, is aroused by means of Yogic practices, so that the Bhujangī can be taken through the six psychic centres within the human body to reach the realisation which leads to release from bondage. We are told that man is in essence "the power-holder of S'iva", 'pure consciousness'—as compared with 'mind and body' which is the manifestation of 'S'iva's Power'—the 'S'akti or Mother'. Therefore, in essence man is of the nature of both S'iva and S'akti. "He is", we are told, "an expression of Power". Kuṇḍalinī-Yoga is the means by which the power within ourselves is raised to its "perfect expression", as Avalon remarks and "is perfect in the sense of unlimited experience". He (the Sādhaka) then attains Bliss.

Kuṇḍalinī-Yoga requires a metaphysical and scientific approach to be made to it. The need to know and understand the darśanas and their implications particularly with reference to Advaita is a great necessity. Woodroffe writes: "The Spirit which is in man is the one Spirit which is in everything and which, as the object of worship, is the Lord (Īśvara) or God. Mind and Matter are many and of many degrees and qualities. Ātma or Spirit as such is the Whole (Pūrṇa) without section (Akhaṇḍa). Mind and matter are parts in that Whole. They are the not-Whole (Apūrṇa) and are the section (Khaṇḍa). Spirit is infinite (Aparicchinna) and formless (Arūpa). Mind and Matter are finite (Paricchinna) and with form (Rūpa). Ātma is unchanged and inactive. Its Power (S'akti) is active and changes in the form of Mind and Matter. Pure consciousness is Cit or Saṃvit. Matter as such is the unconscious. And Mind too is unconscious according to Vedānta. For all that is not the conscious self is the unconscious object. This does not mean that it is unconscious in itself. On the contrary, all is essentially consciousness, but that it is unconscious because it is the object of the conscious self. For mind limits Consciousness so as to enable man to have finite experience. There is no mind without consciousness as its background, though supreme Consciousness is Mindless (Amanah). Where there is no mind (Amanah), there is no limitation. Consciousness remaining in one aspect unchanged changes in its other aspect as active Power which manifests as Mind and Body. Man then is Pure Consciousness (Cit) vehicled by its Power as Mind and Body." (Pp. 20-21).

The Jīva is embodied consciousness. It is the merit of Kuṇḍalinī-Yoga that it helps this embodied consciousness to become aware of its unlimited and undying consciousness. For this Yoga—and Yoga in general—makes it possible for one to transcend human life into the larger and greater one of Being—which is attained by a study of the three states of existence (Avasthātraya). Liberation comes when we realise the source from which we arise. Yoga is the reverse process or return-movement of creation. "The Yoga-process is a return-movement to the Source which is the reverse of the creative movement therefrom. The order of Production is as follows: Buddhi, then Ahaṅkāra, from the latter the Manas, Indriya and Tanmātra and from the last the Bhūta. As the seat of the Source is in the human body the cerebrum in which there is the greater display of Consciousness, the seat of Mind is between the eyebrows and the seats of Matter in the five centres from the throat to the base of the spine. Commencement of the return-movement is made here and the various kinds of Matter are dissolved into one another, and then into Mind and Mind into

Consciousness as described later in Chapter V. To the question whether man can *here and now* attain the supreme state of Bliss, the answer in Yoga is 'yes'." (P. 82).

The processes which help to speed this Yoga on its road to achievements consist of meditation on the mystic formula of seed-letters (mantra), a knowledge of the Six Centres in the human body (Saṭcakranirūpaṇa), and the process of dissolution, known as 'Layakrama'. He who under the special direction of a spiritual guide goes through these stages will attain the highest state of Being. As the author remarks, "Putting aside detail, the main principle appears to be that, when 'wakened', Kuṇḍalinī-S'akti either Herself (or as my friend suggests, in Her eject) ceases to be a static power which sustains the world-consciousness, the content of which is held only so long as She 'sleeps', and, when once set in movement, is drawn to that other static centre in the thousand-petalled lotus (Sahasrāra), which is Herself in union with the S'iva-consciousness or the consciousness of ecstasy beyond the world of forms. When Kuṇḍalinī 'sleeps' man is awake to this world. When She 'awakes' he sleeps—that is, loses all consciousness of the world and enters his causal body. In Yoga he passes beyond to formless Consciousness." (Pp. 313-314).

The *chefs-d'oeuvre* in this book are the two Sanskrit works called 'Saṭ-cakra-Nirūpaṇa' and 'Pāduka pancaka' with commentaries by Kālīcaraṇa . These works are masterly treatises dealing with every detail of this magnificent Yoga, and it is to a great Englishman that we have to be indebted for fixing our attention on their importance in our lives. Woodroffe's translation and notes are all that is to be desired, for it is a real labour of love. In fact, but for this translation no other is available. I hope that all students interested in Indian Occultism will carefully study it and increase their knowledge thereby.

The importance of the Tantras is now well recognised and their significant role in India's thought appreciated.

Verse 52 of Saṭ-cakra-Nirūpaṇa says:

Nītvā tāṁ kulakuṇḍalīm layavaśājjīvena sārdham sudhīr,
mokṣe dhāmanī śudhapadmasadane śaive paresvāmini.
Dhyāyediṣṭaphalapradām bhagavatīm caitanyarūpām parām,
yogindro gurupādapadmayugalālambī samādhau yataḥ.

"The wise and excellent Yogi rapt in ecstasy, and devoted to the Lotus feet of his Guru, should lead Kula-Kuṇḍalī along with Jīva to Her Lord the Para-S'iva in the abode of Liberation within the pure Lotus, and meditate upon Her who grants all desires as the Caitanyarūpa-Bhagavatī. When he thus leads Kula-Kuṇḍalinī, he should make all things absorb into her."

It is the end of this Kuṇḍalinī-Yoga to absorb into its motherly womb the child escaped from the protection of its mother's loving care. Such a sublime philosophy lies behind our Tantras. May the Kuṇḍalinī grant us strength to be re-absorbed into the womb of the Brahman where we rightly and legitimately belong.

—*The Hindu*

SUBTLE CENTRES OF POWER

Dr. C. P. Ramaswami Aiyar

It is remarkable, but also very true, that at a period when we had lost sight of the importance and significance of our own heritage, were busily engaged in westernising ourselves and were, in that process, ignoring the philosophical and practical lessons embedded in our Scriptures, some enthusiastic European scholars brought us to a realisation of the meaning of our past. India owes an immeasurable debt of gratitude to men like Sir William Jones, Colebrooke, Monier Williams, Max Muller and other scholars, German, Russian, French and American, who studied our ancient literature, translated it and commented on it profusely.

Admittedly, however, all of them believed fervidly in the Christian ethos and were somewhat patronising in their attitude towards other faiths and also towards Sanskrit, Tamil and other literatures. There were two conspicuous exceptions, namely, Dr. Annie Besant and Sir John Woodroffe. The latter was, for some time, a Judge of the Calcutta High Court and wrote under the pen-name of Arthur Avalon. All the time that Woodroffe could spare from his judicial duties, he devoted to Hindu philosophy and especially to researches into Tāntric texts and commentaries. He had the good fortune of being actively helped by his wife and he made it a part of his mission to dispel the widely prevalent ignorance regarding the Tāntric S′āstra and to emphasise and to popularise its unique contribution to world-thought.

Controverting, in his *S′akti and S′ākta*, first published about forty years ago, some of the mis-conceptions that were widespread regarding the culture and civilisation of India, he stated:

> "Were I an Indian, I should never surrender my soul to any. The life of India has displayed itself in all activities. It has meditated both as a man of religion and of philosophy but it has also worked in every sphere of activity."

In that collection of essays as well as in the present volume *The Serpent Power*, he asserts that "true life is creative and follows on unity with the world-soul. Man is regarded as a magazine of power. Service of the Devī in any of her aspects is as much worship as are the traditional forms of ritual (Upāsana)." In notable words, the author asserts that union may be had with Reality in Bhukti as in Mukti, in discriminating enjoyment as in liberation, enjoyment being life, the essence of all being. Patriotism was sublimated as a form of worship and Woodroffe affirmed that service of the Mother-form is that aspect of religion which is called true patriotism and which is not in conflict with true humanity.

The present volume is the sixth edition of a work which was published about the same time as *S'akti and S'ākta*. It concerns itself with a description and elucidation of that form of Yoga which concentrates on the manifestation of the Kuṇḍalinī-S'akti. Two Sanskrit works, *Ṣaṭcakra-nirūpaṇa* dealing with the bodily centres of energy, and *Pādukapañcaka* comprising the Guru's function in this form of Yoga, are translated; and following a Bengalee commentary on them, Woodroffe has appended his own commentary and notes and the volume is profusely got up and illustrated. This type of Yoga is also called Laya-Yoga and the work deals with Consciousness as embodied and in its bodiless character. The underlying ideas and the function of S'abda (sound), Varṇa (letters as embodying the secret of sound) and Mantra, are elaborated and the author points out that the creative power of thought is receiving increasing acceptance in the world. Thought, like mind, is described as a power or S′akti and thought as manifested in S′abda or sound and culminating in a Mantra, is dealt with in a special chapter.

The underlying thought of the Indian Scriptures that the Universe is an unfoldment (Sṛṣṭi) from the homogeneous (Mūla-Prakṛti) to the heterogeneous (Vikṛti) and back again to Pralaya (dissolution) is the topic of the chapter entitled "Bodiless Consciousness"; and it is noteworthy that the author cites Prof. Huxley, the celebrated agnostic, as stating: "The manifestations of Cosmic energy alternate between phases of potentiality and phases of explication". Refuting the common mis-representation that Tantra and especially the Kuṇḍalinī-Yoga (termed by him 'The Serpent Fire') have anything to do with the search of gross pleasures or the pursuit of black magic, Woodroffe makes this statement, the truth of which should never be forgotten:

> "The Indian who practises this or any other kind of Yoga, does so, not on account of any interest in occultism or with a desire to practise magic or Nayikasiddhi or similar experiences but because he believes in that practice as part of the quest of the Ātman Brahman".

Indian systems attach paramount importance to Consciousness and its states. Brahmā, Viṣṇu and S′iva are really names for the several functions of the one Universal Consciousness, and Yoga is one of the means employed for the transformation of the lower into higher states of Conscious-sciousness. The object of Kuṇḍalinī-Yoga is to realise the existence of and to stimulate the energy dispersed in various centres in the human body and to concentrate and to bring to a climax the potentialities of those centres which, taken together, are represented in the ideal form of a coiled serpent whose uncoiling results in the manifestation of the Power Reservoir.

In the Introduction to this book occur some sentences which may be said to summarise the author's thesis :

> "All that is manifestis S'akti or Power. Power implies a Power-holder. The Power-holder is S'iva, the Power is S'akti, the great Mother of the Universe."

The Cakras which are stimulated by Mantra and Yoga are, as already stated, subtle centres of operation in the body of the S'aktis or Powers of the various Tattvas or principles which constitute the bodily sheaths. By Layakrama or certain formulated practices, a person utilising the Mantras, Haṭhayoga and the Laya-Yoga, becomes fit for Samādhi.

In the chapter entitled "Theoretical Bases of This Yoga", Kuṇḍalinī-Yoga is described as a partial conversion of the infinite "coiled" Power in man by an awakening of this Kuṇḍalinī-S'akti from a static condition to a dynamic and wakened state. The conclusions of the author are stated in this paradoxical form:

> "When Kuṇḍalinī sleeps, man is awake to this world. When She awakes he sleeps, that is, he loses all consciousness and enters into formless consciousness."

Translations of the two above-mentioned works which follow the introductory portion are clear and illuminating; and although the Tantra Sāstra and especially the forms of Laya-Yoga and Rāja-Yoga described in this book are technical in language and outlook, yet, by his clarity of thought and felicity of expression, Sir John Woodroffe has brought the subject within the comprehension of lay readers and of those unacquainted with the Sanskrit language. Few branches of spiritual striving are as adapted to the needs of the practical man as are certain aspects of the Tantra S'āstra which, it may be noted, makes no distinction between castes and communities, between man and woman and between race and race. The Tantras postulate that physical force (Kriyā S′akti) must be accompanied by disciplined knowledge (Jñāna S′akti) and that the resultant action must be infused by what the author elsewhere terms the Religion of Power—Power directed to right ends and in harmony with the evolving spirit of life.

The public should welcome the appearance of this edition which is a joy to handle and a delight to peruse. Great credit is also due to the publishers, Messrs. Ganesh & Co., for their enterprise in making available to the public editions-de-luxe of the works of persons like Sir John Woodroffe and of other books like the *Saundarya Laharī* which are valuable but not popular in the ordinary sense.

—The Sunday Standard

THE SERPENT POWER

SRI K. GURU DUTT

THIS is the sixth edition of an important Tāntric work edited by Sir John Woodroffe, the great jurist and scholar, under the pen name of Arthur Avalon. Tāntric studies had long been discredited in India as well as the West. It was mainly through his monumental labours that their prestige was restored and their value came to be recognised. He has laid India under a deep debt of gratitude by his fearless championing of one of the most misunderstood aspects of her religion and culture. For many, his writings have proved the harbingers of a revival of faith in the efficacy of *Sādhana* or experimental religion. Practically for the first time in English he has attempted to take spiritualism seriously and to provide its rationale which, although by no means the last word on the subject, is packed with fruitful suggestions. No one who enters this field can advance even a step without paying his tribute of admiration to this courageous pioneer who made himself something of an intellectual out-caste among his own people by venturing into a region which for long had been held to be intellectually 'untouchable'.

This book is a description and explanation of the *Kuṇḍalinī* S'akti, and the *Sādhana* or practice connected with its development, which occupies a prominent place in the scheme of the *Tantra Sāstra.* The process is technically described as *S'aṭ-cakra-bheda* or piercing of the six centres (*Cākras*) or lotuses (*Padmās*) by the agency of *Kuṇḍalinī S'akti.* The Supreme Power residing in the human body is here symbolised as the Goddess (*Devī*), *Kuṇḍalinī* envisaged as a tiny coiled serpent reposing in the lowest body-centre, the *Mūlādhāra*, at the base of the spinal column, until she is aroused and made to traverse six centres or *Cakras* and ultimately reaches the *Sahasrāra Cakra*, resulting in the consummation of ultimate bliss. Of course it cannot be sufficiently emphasised here that actual practice of any form of *Sādhana* requires initiation and competent instruction from a Master at every step. All that books like this can do is to rouse and feed the initial interest, and to provide that background of comprehension without which all practice degenerates into mere mechanism.

The originals of two Sanskrit works with commentaries *viz.* *Ṣaṭ-cakra-Nirūpaṇam* and the smaller *Pāduka Pañcakam* comprise one-third of this book. An English translation of these two works with the main verses transliterated in Roman script together with elaborate notes and explanatory material take up a similar part of this work. The editor's principal contribution is an exhaustive and masterly Introduction covering over 300 pages which provides an ample perspective and background for the whole subject, and deals among other things with the nature of consciousness as bodiless and as embodied, *Mantra* or articulate power, and the centres or lotuses (*Cakra* or *Padma*), and the practical as well as with the theoretical basis of this *Yoga*. Valuable English and Sanskrit Indexes form a feature of this work along with coloured plates depicting the several *Cakras*, as also photographic blocks illustrating the *Yogāsanas*. The book is sumptuously got up and does credit to the enterprise of the Publishers who have done a great service to the country by bringing out a series of works dealing with esoteric aspects of Indian religion and philosophy, which would otherwise have remained in obscurity. The first edition of this book was published forty years ago by M/s. Luzac and Co., London, and had a more rapid sale than was expected. The second edition which was greatly revised and enlarged was brought out by the present Publishers. That the work has now run into the sixth edition is an augury of the increasing tempo of interest in the more recondite aspects of Indian religious philosophy and *Sādhana*.

It would be a mistake to think that this form of *Sādhana* is of comparatively recent origin. The *Nādi* symbolism which, as it were, provides the soil in which this form of *Yoga* is rooted goes back to the earliest Upaniṣads. There are several later *Yogic* Upaniṣads which exclusively deal with this topic. It is broached in some of the Purāṇas or other celebrated works like the *Saundarya Lahari* (attributed to S'ri S'ankarācārya) a splendid edition of which was recently brought out by the present Publishers. The theoretical background which forms the last section of the Introduction covers over 60 pages and treats the subject in all its aspects. It would not be possible within the compass of a short review to go into any of these matters. After all it has to be borne in mind, as the learned Editor has often stressed, that the value of any form of *Sādhana* does not lie in its antiquity, or in the greatness of the names associated with tradition, or even the ethical accompaniments, but mainly in its practical efficacy. The crucial and only test is whether the *Sādhana* leads to *Siddhi* (fulfilment) or not. Or in common language 'the proof of the pudding is in the eating'. In general, it may be said that apart from those familiar aspects of religion and philosophy which are commonly acknowledged, it is beyond doubt that there are occult or hidden regions and in which the investigations made by the ancients would stand us moderns in very good stead if only we would treat them with reverence as worthy of study, instead of discarding them as rank superstitions, following the lead of half-baked foreign scholars and their intellectual progeny in this country. Even in our own time, Masters like S'ri Rāmakrishna Paramahamsa have tested in their own experience the veracity and genuineness of such things. The spectacular advances made in the physical sciences should not blind us to the fact that the psychical experimental sciences had made very great progress in our land in the past, and that we possess an innate aptitude (*Saṁskāra*) for their restoration and development if only we wish to do so. Towards such a desirable end, publications like the present help immensely.

— *Vedanta Kesari*

NEW

VEDIC SYMBOLISM

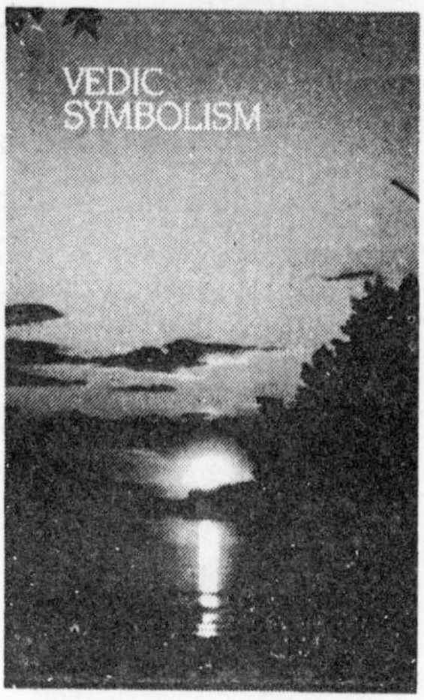

by Sri Aurobindo
compiled by Sri. M.P. Pandit

$6.95; 122 pp.; paper; ISBN: 0-941524-30-2

The value of the Rig Veda as a guidebook to spiritual practice has been obscured due to the heavy veil of symbols used by the Rishis to hide their meaning from the uninitiated. Sri Aurobindo, through many years of research and sadhana, was able to unlock the secret of the veda and give us the key to the symbolic system of the Vedic Rishis.

"Vedic Symbolism" introduces the major vedic concepts and reveals their esoteric sense. Sri Aurobindo's work has given the study of the Rig Veda new relevance and has made the imagery of the Veda reveal its hidden meaning. It is an important contribution to the vedic literature.

Yoga Books Authored by SRI M.P. PANDIT

YOGA OF WORKS

$7.95; 186 pp.; paper; ISBN: 0-941524-21-3

YOGA OF KNOWLEDGE

$7.95; 280 pp.; paper; ISBN: 0-941524-23-X

YOGA OF LOVE

$3.95; 104 pp.; paper; ISBN: 0-941524-16-7

YOGA OF SELF PERFECTION

$7.95; 308 pp.; paper; ISBN: 0-941524-20-5

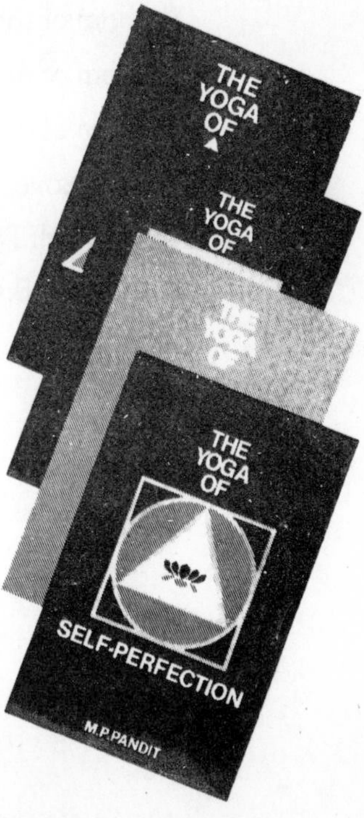

This series of books systematically reviews the "Synthesis of Yoga" of Sri Aurobindo, chapter by chapter and presents the essence of the yogic process in a warm and readable way. The "Yoga of Works" explores the processes of "Karma Yoga". The "Yoga of Knowledge" presents the way of the intellect, developing through concentration, meditation and silencing of the mind. The "Yoga of Love" reveals the path of the heart, through love, devotion, and "bhakti". Finally, in the "Yoga of Self Perfection", Panditji extrapolates on the unique contribution Sri Aurobindo has made to the practice of yoga, the integration of spirituality and the life of material, physical, vital and mental perfection into a unified science of self perfection.

OTHER TITLES BY M. P. PANDIT

Bases of Tantra Sadhana	2.00
Dhyana (Meditation)	1.95
Dictionary of Sri Aurobindo's Yoga	11.95
How Do I Begin?	3.00
How Do I Proceed?	3.00
Kundalini Yoga	4.95
Occult Lines Behind Life	7.95
Spiritual Life: Theory and Practice	7.95
Yoga for the Modern Man	4.00
Sri Aurobindo and His Yoga	6.95
Upanishads: Gateways of Knowledge	9.95
Vedic Deities	7.95
Vedic Symbolism (compiler)	6.95
Wisdom of the Upanishads (compiler)	7.95
Wisdom of the Gita, 1st Series	9.95
Wisdom of the Veda	7.95
Yoga of Love	3.95
Yoga of Self Perfection	7.95
Yoga of Works	7.95
Yoga of Knowledge	7.95